Contents

Preface

Global health in the network of international research collaborations
5 years Institute for Research in International Assistance (IRIA)

Dear activists for global health, dear colleagues,

The Institute for Research in International Assistance (IRIA) celebrates its five-year anniversary in May 2023, a good opportunity to look back at the various collaborative projects and activities and to have an outlook to the coming five years. Since its foundation, IRIA followed up on the idea of organizing scientific partnerships to support and further research and development of health and well-being in general, health care systems in particular and address supra-national global health questions, challenges and initiatives. Some projects, especially with Eastern European partners are based on projects of the Koch-Mechnikov-Forum, an initiative to support German-Eastern-European partnerships in health, originally with Russia as main partner country, since February 2022 without.

IRIA has several formats of activity:
- Scientific and/or praxis-oriented collaborative projects, mainly bilateral and third-party-funded
- Exchange programs for students, young researchers, senior scientists, mediated by several exchange organizations, including DAAD, Institut für Auslandsbeziehungen (ifa), International Sustainability Academy (ISA), Engagement Global (asa programm) etc.
- Scientific meetings, especially serial symposia like the symposium on the occasion of World Tuberculosis Day each March or the International Young Researchers' Symposium (IYRS) as part of the World Health Summit satellite program
- Education and training via seminars, workshops, webinars or international summer schools

Indonesia is already a cooperation country for German development cooperation. So far, the partnership has focused particularly on climate protection and sustainable development, promotion of the private sector and good governance. Furthermore, as an emerging economy, Indonesia is a partner for triangular cooperation with developing countries.

Akkon University of Human Sciences with its Institute for Research in International Assistance (IRIA) sees Indonesia as the healthcare system of an emerging market and is now taking another step in deepening development cooperation with a pioneering Indonesia project: "Promotion of Health Sciences in Indonesia & the German-Indonesian Partnership in Research & Teaching in Public Health". With Mohammadiyah University in Indonesia, a new promising partnership was established in autumn 2022. In concrete terms, this initially involves two focal points:

1. Joint teaching & preparation of a German-Indonesian Master program in Public & Global Health, which combines medical and health content with social and political science approaches. The target audiences are physicians, paramedics, nurses, other non-medical fields
2. Research projects on infectious diseases, NCDs (Non-Communicable Diseases), poverty-related diseases, social determinants of diseases, health system analysis and strengthening

The encouragement for this new cooperation came not least from the involvement of Indonesian experts and scientists in Akkon/IRIA symposia and forums, including the Young Researchers' Symposium (IYRS) in October 2022. This event is one of IRIA's overarching formats dedicated to promoting young researchers.

To honor the new partnership with Indonesia, the decision matured to summarize the results of the IYRS in October 2022 in this new focus publication, the sixth edition of Akkon Schriftenreihe.

This IYRS assembled 21 projects of young colleagues dealing with an amazing range of topics and research questions in global health. The presented projects ranged from clinical to public health research questions and from the Caribbean to Africa, Eastern Europe, India and also Indonesia. Contents and scientific discussions were of very high quality.

We would like to thank all contributors, their supervisors, their respective institutions and also sponsors for supporting their works which now form an impressive and insightful overview of various projects dedicated to improve health in an changing and challenging environment.

We are looking forward to continuing and deepening our collaborative work and wish you joy and inspiration while reading.

Timo Ulrichs & Gaby Feldmann
Head of Institute of Research in International Assistance (IRIA) / Akkon University

#Preface

Global cooperation at eye level

We congratulate IRIA to their anniversary and their excellent work during the past 5 years. ifa – Institut für Auslandsbeziehungen champions freedom in art, research, and civil society worldwide, bringing together people who are committed to an open society. It creates analogue and digital spaces for encounter, exchange, negotiation, and co-creation. ifa lends a voice to activists, artists, scholars, and scientists, promotes cooperation, and increasingly pursues its goals.

One of our funding programmes, CrossCulture Programme (CCP), supports professionals and committed volunteers from the cultural, educational, scientific, artistic and medial sectors to work together. Focal points of the programme are human rights, sustainable development and policy-making, therefore the collaboration with institutions and persons working for the promotion of education, gender equality and health is vital to us – especially in the framework of feminist foreign policies. Women and LGBTIQA have special needs when it comes to health services that need to be acknowledged. Examples are infant mortality, menstrual health and hygiene or the need for special treatments of transgender people or stereotypes when it comes to HIV.

The Akkon University of Applied Sciences / IRIA has been a host organisation of CCP since 2018. CCP Fellows have benefited from Akkon's resources and connections as well as contributed to the research and network of the University. CCP Fellow Rhondemo Kikon from Northern India e.g. focussed on health care for vulnerable groups during his Fellowship with Akkon, while Dr. Roodjmie Nazaire from Haiti dealt with the topics of tuberculosis and gender equality. Indonesian Fellow Hera Susanti researched reproductive health and rights in Indonesia and shared her knowledge with students from Akkon University.

These forms of collaboration between global partners are essential for the solution of worldwide challenges. ifa is looking forward to the upcoming 5 years of fruitful collaboration with IRIA.

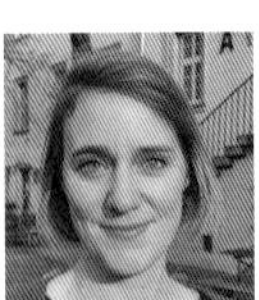

Anne Kruse
Head of Division | CrossCulture Programme
www.ifa.de

Congratulations to IRIA to their fifth anniversary and great work. We value the partnership of IRIA with Engagement Global/ASA program and are looking forward to future cooperation.

Personal encounters, exchange and engagement are at the core of the ASA program. For more than 60 years, ASA has brought together motivated students and young people with vocational training from Germany and countries in Africa, Asia, Latin America and Southeastern Europe to work together in order to find solutions for global challenges.

In cooperation with partner institutions around the world, Engagement Global awards 280 scholarships each year to young people to participate in the ASA program. They are involved in more than 140 projects working on a broad range of sustainable development topics. A special feature is that the partner organizations propose the projects themselves. The Akkon University of Applied Sciences / IRIA has been a valued project partner for several years now. Working on women empowerment and global health, the projects have made an important impact towards driving sustainable development and enabling students worldwide to work together. In this way, Engagement Global and its partners make an important contribution to development education.

More information:
https://asa.engagement-global.de
https://www.instagram.com/asaprogramm

#01.1 Global
Smoking behaviour in adolescents aged 13–14 years in the World: Literature Review

Gandi Puad Pratama, Erliga Nur Hikmah, Ghozali, Nida Amalia, Sri Sunarti, Kresna Febriyanto

Smoking behavior in adolescents is a bad behavior and has a negative impact. As many as 34.7% of teenagers in Indonesia who are over 10 years old are smokers. The purpose of this literature study is to find out from existing literature sources what are the determinants of smoking behavior in adolescents. To answer this, it is necessary to summarize some published results from research on smoking behavior in adolescents.

METHOD. The method used in this research is literature review. This study uses several relevant literature search sources in the database, including Scopus, PubMed, Sciuredirect, and the Google Scholar search engine. Searches for articles in English use keywords: determinants, smoking, youth, Demographic and health survey (DHS), while searches for Indonesian-language journals use keywords: keywords: determinants, smoking, youth, Demographics and health surveys (SDK).

RESULTS. There are ten articles which state that smoking behavior can be related to age, education level, health insurance, employment, religion, area of residence, frequency of use of radio, television and newspapers.

CONCLUSION AND IMPLICATIONS. The lower the self-concept in adolescents, the higher the smoking behavior. This is because a low self-concept causes adolescents to be easily influenced by their surroundings.

KEYWORDS. Smoking, Adolescents, Demographic and health survey (SDK).

Smoking behavior in adolescents is a bad behavior and has a negative impact. A total of 34.7% of adolescents in Indonesia aged over 10 years are smokers. The purpose of this literature study is to find out from the existing literature sources what are the determinants of smoking behavior in adolescents. To answer this, it is necessary to summarize some of the published results of research on smoking behavior in adolescents.

METHODS. The method used in this research is literature review. This literature uses several sources of relevant literature searches in the database, including Scopus, PubMed, Sciuredirect, and the Google Scholar search engine. Search for English articles using keywords: determinant, smoking, youth, Demographic and health survey (DHS), while searching for Indonesian language journals use keywords: determinant, smoking, youth, Demographics and health surveys (SDK).

RESULTS. There are ten articles which state that smoking behavior can be related to age, education level, health insurance, occupation, religion, area of residence, frequency of use of radio, television and newspapers.

CONCLUSIONS AND IMPLICATIONS. The lower the self-concept in adolescents, the higher the smoking behavior. This is because low self-concept causes adolescents to be easily influenced by their surroundings.

KEYWORDS. Smoking, Adolescents, Demographic and health surveys (SDK).

1. PRELIMINARY. The trend of smoking among young people is a global problem, and the effects of smoking are contributing to increased mortality worldwide (Knaappila, Marttunen, Fröjd, Lindberg, &KaltalaHeino, 2019). According to WHO (2015), the percentage of the world's population that consumes tobacco is 57% of the population of Asia and Australia, 14% of the population of Eastern Europe and the Soviet Union, 12% of the American population, 9% of the population of Western Europe and 8% of the population of the Middle East. as well as Africa. Meanwhile ASEAN is an area with 10% of all world smokers and 20% of global causes of death due to tobacco (Alamsyah, 2017). Smoking cases occur mostly in upper-middle income and low income countries, including Indonesia (WHO, 2017).

A study by(Tang et al., 2018)found that smoking is not only a health problem, but also has a significant impact on socioeconomic status, quality of life, and welfare of a country.

Based on a study by the Data and Information Center of the Indonesian Ministry of Health, the prevalence of smoking by sex shows that the prevalence of smoking among adolescent boys is 66% higher than 6.7% (Ministry of Health, 2018). In Asia, data from the Asean Tobacco Atlas 2018 shows 19.8% of Indonesians are classified as first-time smokers among adolescents aged 13-15 years, with an average of 35.3% (Lian &Doroteo, 2018). In Indonesia, the 2018 Basic Health Research data shows that the prevalence of smoking in adolescents aged 10 to 18 years has increased from 7.2% in 2013 to 9.1% in 2018, indicating a significant increase among adolescents (Ministry of Health, 2018) .

Demographic characteristic of study participants in the Timor-leste GYTS 2009,

Characteristics	Total N (%)
Age (years)	
<15	817 (51.0 %)
15 +	798 (49.0 %)
Gender	
Boys	752 (47.0 %)
Girls	849 (53.0 %)
Education level (grades)	
Grade 1	445 (27.0 %)
Grade 2	732 (45.0 %)
Grade 3	439 (27.0 %)
Currently smoking	
Yes	667 (51.0 %)
No	649 (49.0 %)

#01.1 Global
Smoking behaviour in adolescents aged 13–14 years in the World: Literature Review

Tobacco use during adolescence is associated with adverse health effects later in life. Adolescence is the most critical period in life and is accompanied by rapid physical, psychological and emotional development and changes, and smoking at this age can be more dangerous for adolescent health by increasing the risk of developing chronic diseases (So and Yeo 2015). In addition, tobacco also has a negative impact on public health and the economy. Smoking is considered a disease listed at level ten of the International Classification of Diseases (ICD-10; F17), so it deserves attention.

Various measures have been implemented to reduce the prevalence of smoking, one of which is by providing warning illustrations on tobacco packaging. Despite implementing a tobacco use cessation strategy, the reduction in smoking prevalence has not been significant.

The purpose of this literature review is to find out from existing literature sources what are the determinants of smoking behavior in adolescents. To answer this, it is necessary to summarize some published results from research on smoking behavior in adolescents. We hope that the results of this literature review can be a source of additional literature and information about the factors that influence smoking behavior in adolescents.

2. METHODOLOGY. The method used in this research is literature review. This study uses several relevant literature search sources in the database, including Scopus, PubMed, Sciuredirect, and the Google Scholar search engine. Searches for articles in English use keywords: determinants, smoking, youth, Demographic and health survey (DHS), while searches for Indonesian-language journals use keywords: keywords: determinants, smoking, youth, Demographics and health surveys (SDK).

This study aims to determine what factors influence smoking behavior in adolescents from various sources. This research was conducted to seek a systematic approach using inclusion criteria. Literature searches are limited from 2015 to 2022 with articles in Indonesian and English. Literature searches using the Scopus, PubMed, Sciuredirect and Google Scholar Search Engine databases were carried out by researchers with keywords resulting in 4,170 articles. Then classification, adjustment of title and year of publication was carried out, and 170 articles were obtained. After that, abstracts and full texts were selected for the ninety-eight articles. Final results adjusted for inclusion and exclusion criteria, resulting in twelve articles including author, year, title, design, sample, variable,

3. RESULTS. The results of the literature review resulted in 10 reviews that were included in the terms and inclusion criteria, namely (Nketiah-Amponsah et al., 2018), (Tang et al., 2018), (Abdulrahim &

Jawad, 2018), (Magati et al., 2018), (Kelishadi et al., 2016), (Zaborskis & Sirvyte, 2015), (Okagua, Opara, & Alex-Hart, 2016), (Ribeiro Sarmento & Yehadji, 2016), (Doku, Acacio-Claro, Koivusilta, & Rimpelä, 2019), (Nagrath et al., 2019) From ten literatures, it appears that the factors that influence smoking can be related to age, education, health insurance, employment, religion, place of residence, frequency of use of radio, television and newspapers.

4. DISCUSSION. Overall, the results of this study indicate that smoking is related to gender, age, employment status, education level, wealth status, area of residence, access to media, adolescents whose parents smoke have a higher risk of smoking behavior and lack of understanding of the impact bad cigarettes from smoking. Adolescence is counted as the age when trying new things and taking risks (Ministry of Health, 2016).

Prevalence Of Cigarrete Smoking By Gender, 2003–2014.

Smokes cigarette	2003 GDHS		2008 GDHS		2014 GDHS	
	Male	Female	Male	Female	Male	Female
No	90.95	99.91	92.69	99.83	95.22	99.93
Yes	9.05	0.09	7.31	0.17	4.78	0.07

Column percentages reported. Source: Computed by authors from the 2003, 2008 & 2014 GDHS

Adolescence exposes some teenagers to friends and the environment that can shape their personality, one of which is smoking behavior (Efendi, Aidah, Has, Lindayani, &Reisenhofer, 2019).

Association between each demoghraphic variable and current smoking status among in-school students in Timor-Leste (an estimate of smoking rate is 51.0%)

Characteristics	Current smoking status		P-value
	Yes	No	
	N (%)	N (%)	
Age			
<15	299 (46.0 %)	365 (54.0 %)	<0.05
15+	351 (57.0 %)	270 (43.0 %)	
Gender			
Boys	380 (59.0 %)	177 (41.0 %)	<0.05
Girls	236 (28.0 %)	457 (72.0 %)	
Education level (grades)			
Grade 1	175 (53.0 %)	156 (47.0 %)	>0.05
Grade 2	292 (49.0 %)	304 (51.0 %)	
Grade 3	178 (50.0 %)	180 (50.0 %)	

The rate of smoking behavior is closely related to the level of education, research conducted in Ethiopia states that someone with a higher education has a 44% lower likelihood of smoking compared to someone who has no education (Guliani, Gamtessa, & Çule, 2019). Access to good information makes the desire to smoke high because teenagers can easily obtain information so they have a great desire to smoke. (Rudi, Masan, & Kwureh, 2017).

In addition to these factors smoking behavior in adolescents can be related to parents who smoke and this study recommends holding family discussions about the harmful effects of smoking; smoking in areas such as schools, public places and homes; and cigarette ads on billboards (Ribeiro Sarmento & Yehadji, 2016). Other studies have also found that smoking in adolescents is associated with families experiencing divorce which causes an increase in smoking habits and low academic achievement. This study recommends that the orientation of adolescent education through health education can be the main strategy for preventing adolescent smoking, counseling on smoking cessation to improve health equality , emphasized (Doku et al., 2019). Research from literature reviews has several weaknesses, including most of the articles derived from quantitative studies so they cannot explain the causes and effects of smoking behavior in adolescent boys.

The implications of the research that has been done need to be adjusted to the policies in each country. Most of the research also uses secondary data, so that the search for articles is limited by variables that are relevant to smoking behavior. The difference found from the studies that have been conducted is that smoking behavior in adolescents can be influenced by several factors, including internal factors and external factors. However, in Indonesia research on the factors that influence smoking behavior in male adolescents using national secondary data from the 2017 Indonesian Demographic and Health Survey on Adolescent Reproductive Health (SDKI KRR) has never been studied.

5. CONCLUSION. Smoking behavior illustrated in this study includes gender, age, employment status, education level, wealth status, area of residence, media access, adolescents with parents who smoke and lack of knowledge about the effects of smoking. Prevention of smoking behavior needs to be adapted to the characteristics of adolescents who smoke, so that information and actions can be targeted and effective in reducing smoking behavior in male adolescents. Cigarette consumption needs to be limited by prohibiting sales by and for teenagers as well as packaging and labeling of scary images caused by smoking. Concrete steps need to be taken related to government policies, one of which is controlling the selling price by increasing cigarette excise duty every year so that not just anyone can consume cigarettes.—

BIBLIOGRAPHY

Abdulrahim, S., & Jawad, M. (2018). Socioeconomic differences in smoking in Jordan, Lebanon, Syria, and Palestine: A cross-sectional analysis of national surveys. PLoS ONE, 13(1), e0189829. • Aho, H., Koivisto, AM, Paavilainen, E., &Joronen, K. (2019). The relationship between peer relations, self-rated health and smoking behavior in secondary vocational schools. Nurs Open, 6(3), 754-764. doi:10.1002/nop2.260. • Efendi, F., Aidah, FN, Has, EMM, Lindayani, L., &Reisenhofer, S. (2019). Determinants of smoking behavior among young males in rural Indonesia. International Journal of Adolescent Medicine and Health. doi:10.1515/ijamah-2019-0040. • Guliani, H., Gamtessa, S., &Çule, M. (2019). Factors affecting tobacco smoking in Ethiopia: Evidence from the demographic and health surveys. BMC Public Health, 19(1). doi:10.1186/s12889-019- 7200-8. • Kelishadi, R., Heshmat, R., Shahsanai, A., Djalalinia, S., Motlagh, ME, Keikha, M., . . . Asayesh, H. (2016). Determinants of tobacco and hookah smoking in a nationally representative sample of Iranian children and adolescents: the Caspian-IV study. Iranian Red Crescent Medical Journal, 18(8). • Ministry of Health. (2018a). Riskesdas 2018 results. In: Ministry of Health Health Research and Development Agency. • Ministry of Health. (2018b). Indonesia Health Profile 2017. In MKY drg. Rudy Kurniawan, SKM, M.Si Boga Hardhana, S.Si, MM Tanti Siswanti, SKM, M.Kes (Ed.). • Magati, P., Drope, J., Mureithi, L., & Lencucha, R. (2018). Socio-economic and demographic determinants of tobacco use in Kenya: Findings from the Kenya demographic and health survey 2014. Pan African Medical Journal, 30, 1–10. https://doi.org/10.11604/pamj.2018.30.166.14771 • Nagrath, D., Mathur, MR, Gupta, R., & Zodpey, SP (2019). Socio-demographic and socioeconomic differences in tobacco use prevalence among Indian youth. Preventive Medicine Reports, 14(June 2018), 21–24. https://doi.org/10.1016/j.pmedr.2019.100832 • Nketiah-Amponsah, E., Afful-Mensah, G., & Ampaw, S. (2018). Determinants of cigarette smoking and smoking intensity among adult males in Ghana. BMC Public Health, 18(1), 1–10. https://doi.org/10.1186/s12889-018-5872-0 • Ribeiro Sarmento, D., & Yehadji, D. (2016). An analysis of global youth tobacco survey for developing a comprehensive national smoking policy in Timor-Leste. BMC Public Health, 16(1), 1–7. https://doi.org/10.1186/s12889-016-2742-5 • Tang, S., Bishwajit, G., Luba, TR, & Yaya, S. (2018). Prevalence of smoking among men in Ethiopia and Kenya: A cross-sectional study. International Journal of Environmental Research and Public Health, 15(6). https://doi.org/10.3390/ijerph15061232 • Zaborskis, A., & Sirvyte, D. (2015). Familial determinants of current smoking among adolescents of Lithuania: A cross-sectional survey 2014. BMC Public Health, 15(1), 1–12. https://doi.org/10.1186/s12889 015 2230 3

AUTHORS

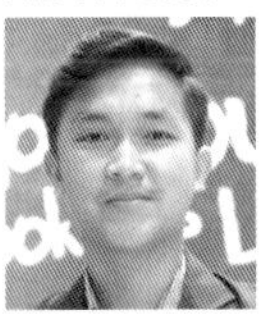

Gandi Puad Pratama
Faculty of Public Health | UMKT; Indonesia | E-mail: gandipuadpratama07@umkt.ac.id

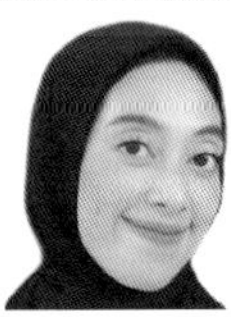

Erliga Nur Hikmah
Faculty of Public Health | UMKT; Indonesia |
E-mail: erliga05@umkt.ac.id

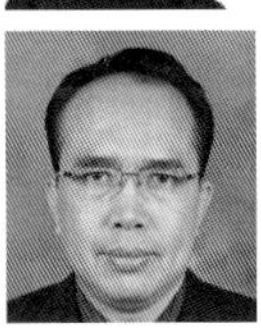

Ghozali
Faculty of Public Health | UMKT; Indonesia | E-mail: gm760@umkt.ac.id

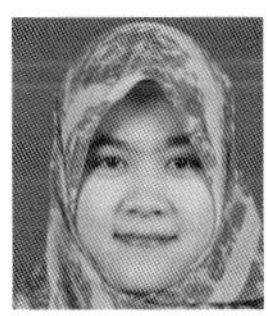

Nida Amalia
Faculty of Public Health | UMKT; Indonesia |
E-mail: na844@umkt.ac.id

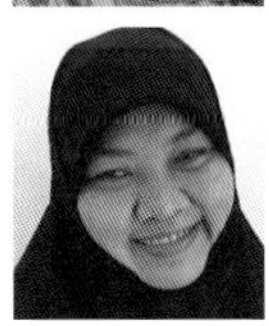

Sri Sunarti
Faculty of Public Health | UMKT; Indonesia |
E-mail: ss678@umkt.ac.id

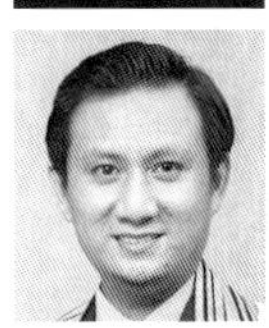

Kresna Febriyanto
Faculty of Public Health | UMKT; Indonesia |
E-mail: kresna.kesmas@umkt.ac.id

Universitas Muhammadiyah Kalimantan Timur (UMKT)
Samarinda, Indonesia
E-mail: gandipuadpratama07@gmail.com | nidaamalia@umkt.ac.id

#01.2 Global
Acute malnutrition: Why food insecurity during emergencies should not be overlooked

Fekri Dureab, Raof Al-Waziza

Acute malnutrition or wasting refers to a child's low weight for height. Rapid weight loss or failure to gain weight leads to acute malnutrition. Globally, there are more than 45.4 million under-five children acutely malnourished, 13.6 million of them suffer from severe acute malnutrition[1]. Wasting contributes to nearly 1 million under-five children's deaths annually worldwide[2]. According to UNICEF's conceptual framework of malnutrition, inadequate food intake and recurrent infectious morbidity represent the immediate causes of undernutrition. Underlying causes are categorized in three main themes; food, practice and health services[3].

Nutrition in crisis refers to a situation where individuals or communities lack access to adequate and/or nutritious food. This can occur during natural disasters, armed conflicts, economic downturns, and other emergency situations. In the humanitarian conditions resulting from disasters and wars, supplies are cut off, access to food is reduced, and health services deteriorate, which causes an increase in cases of severe acute malnutrition. Consequently, morbidity and mortality increase among vulnerable groups, especially among under-five children. As the conflict continues in Ukraine, access to food and clean drinking water, proper sanitation as well as healthcare have been disturbed. Moreover, livelihoods, markets, and supply chains have been severely affected. These factors contribute in adding extra pressure on families to meet their immediate food needs. According to an assessment conducted by the World Food Programme (WFP), one-third of Ukraine's households were found to be food insecure[4]. In fact, several countries are currently facing a food security emergency due to the macroeconomic crisis as a result of the Russian-Ukraine conflict that amplified the inflation rate in many countries around the world. For instance, in Sudan, the national inflation rate increased to 144 percent in 2020 and devastated purchasing power of local people[5]. Natural crises and pandemics can exacerbate the situation of food insecurity. For instance, the COVID-19 pandemic has had a significant impact on global food systems, leading to disruptions in food supply chains, increased food prices, and reduced purchasing power for many people, which in turn has contributed to an increase in malnutrition in some populations. This is especially true in low- and middle-income countries, where the majority of the world's food scarcity and malnourished people live. Additionally, the pandemic has hindered access to healthcare as well as to preventive and curative nutrition services, exacerbating the problem[6].

Malnutrition in crisis situations can be caused by a combination of factors, including limited access to adequate food, poor sanitation and hygiene, and increased risk of infectious diseases. In such situations, the population is particularly vulnerable and the consequences of malnutrition can be severe, including increased morbidity and mortality. In particular, children, pregnant, breastfeeding women, and the elderly are more likely subjected to suffer from acute malnutrition. Malnutrition can impair the immune system and make an individual more susceptible to infections and diseases[7]. People who are malnourished, especially those with deficiencies in vitamins and minerals, may have weakened immune systems, making them more susceptible to infections and increasing their risk of severe illness and death. Recently, during the COVID-19 pandemic, several proofs showed that malnutrition could have long-term effects on the severity of COVID-19 where it can affect lung function, making it more difficult for the body to cope with the respiratory stress of COVID-19. In some cases, malnutrition can also lead to comorbidities, such as heart disease and diabetes, that increase the risk of severe illness from COVID-19, the mortality among patients COVID-19 with malnutrition reached to 10 times more likely as compared to those who were well-nourished[8,9].

CONCLUSION. Malnutrition, including undernutrition and micronutrient deficiencies, can have serious health consequences, and can be especially harmful to under-five children, pregnant and lactating women, and the elderly. Managing acute malnutrition cases and providing food assistance is unlikely to lead to a lasting solution, unless other causes are addressed at the same time such as proper management of underlying diseases, community awareness enhancement about exclusive breastfeeding, best feeding practice, hygiene and general improvement of the national economy. In crisis situations, the provision of emergency food assistance, as well as interventions to improve food security and nutrition, are crucial to protecting the health and well-being of affected populations. To address this issue, it is important to strengthen food systems, improve access to nutrition services, and provide targeted support to populations most at risk of malnutrition.—

REFERENCES

1 United Nations Children's Fund (UNICEF), World Health Organization (WHO) & International Bank for Reconstruction and Development/The World Bank. Levels and trends in child malnutrition: key findings of the 2021 edition of the joint child malnutrition estimates. , <https://www.who.int/publications/i/item/9789240025257> (2021). **2** Kambale, R. M. & Francisca, I. N. Optimising the management of acute malnutrition. The Lancet Global Health 10, e453-e454, doi:10.1016/S2214-109X(22)00087-0 (2022). **3** UNICEF. UNICEF Conceptual Framework on Maternal and Child Nutrition, <https://www.unicef.org/media/113291/file/UNICEF%20Conceptual%20Framework.pdf> (2021). **4** WFP. Ukraine Food Security Report <https://docs.wfp.org/api/documents/WFP-0000139511/download/?_ga=2.39149731.1026792365.1670853611-829821828.1670853611> (2022). **5** Abu-Manga, M., Al-Jawaldeh, Ayoub, Qureshi, Abdul B., Ali, Amira M.E., Pizzol, Damiano, Dureab, Fekri. Nutrition Assessment of Under-Five Children in Sudan: Tracking the Achievement of the Global Nutrition Targets. Children 8, 363, doi:https://doi.org/10.3390/children8050363 (2021). **6** Dasgupta, S. & Robinson, E. J. Z. Impact of COVID-19 on food insecurity using multiple waves of high frequency household surveys. Sci Rep-Uk 12, 1865, doi:10.1038/s41598-022-05664-3 (2022). **7** Schaible, U. E. & Kaufmann, S. H. E. Malnutrition and Infection: Complex Mechanisms and Global Impacts. Plos Med 4, e115, doi:10.1371/journal.pmed.0040115 (2007). **8** Abate, S. M., Chekole, Y. A., Estifanos, M. B., Abate, K. H. & Kabthymer, R. H. Prevalence and outcomes of malnutrition among hospitalized COVID-19 patients: A systematic review and meta-analysis. Clinical Nutrition ESPEN 43, 174-183, doi:https://doi.org/10.1016/j.clnesp.2021.03.002 (2021). **9** Kurtz, A. et al. Long-term effects of malnutrition on severity of COVID-19. Sci Rep-Uk 11, 14974, doi:10.1038/s41598-021-94138-z (2021).

AUTHORS

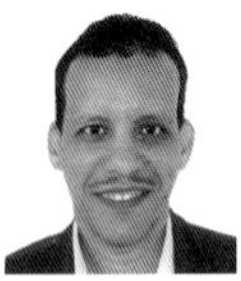

Dr. Fekri Dureab
Research Associate Institute for Research in International Assistance (IRIA), Akkon Hochschule für Humanwissenschaften, Berlin, Germany & Heidelberg Institute of Global Health, Medical School, Ruprecht-Karls-University, Heidelberg, Germany
E-mail: fekri.dureab@iria.akkon-hochschule.de

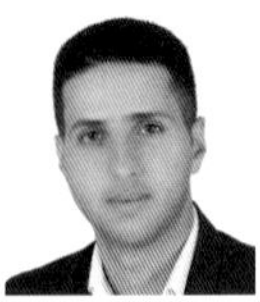

Raof Al-Waziza
Research Associate, Institute for Research in International Assistance (IRIA), Akkon Hochschule für Humanwissenschaften, Berlin, Germany
E-mail: raof.alwaziza@iria.akkon-hochschule.de

#02 Antigua
Combating Childhood Obesity in Antigua and Barbuda
Nana Konadu-Asare, Ashleigh Bates, Leslie Walwyn

INTRODUCTION. The World Health Organization (WHO) defines obesity as "the abnormal or excessive fat accumulation that impairs health". According to the WHO, in 2016 1.9 billion or 39% of adults 18 years or older were identified as obese globally.[1] In 2019, 38.2 million children under 5 were identified as obese and a total of 340 million children and adolescents from ages 5–19 were considered overweight or obese.1 Obesity has tripled worldwide in prevalence since 1975 with an exponential growth pattern seen in childhood obesity.[1] The effects of obesity have significantly affected Caribbean countries, with 140 million people and one in three children considered obese.[1]
Antigua and Barbuda (AB) rank third for obesity in the Caribbean region with a total prevalence of 31% impacting both adults and children based on the Pan American Health Organization (PAHO) data.[2] In addition, according to the WHO, the prevalence of childhood obesity in Antigua is 38.2% with 26.7% of children identified as overweight and 11.5% identified as obese.[3]
Obesity is tied to cardiovascular disease, diabetes, musculoskeletal disorders, cancers, depression, and low self-esteem.[4] In addition to health consequences, obesity poses a financial burden on the economy. Thus, the aim of this paper is to identify the social, economic, environmental risk factors and consequences of childhood obesity in AB. Furthermore, discuss proposed solutions for better prevention and management.

ANTIGUA AND BARBUDA. AB is a twin-island identified as a small island developing state (or SIDS) in the Eastern Caribbean[5] and relies heavily on external resources for sustainability. The population consists of approximately 100,000 people with 97% living in Antigua. The Gross Domestic Product (GDP) is $1.47B US Dollars ranking AB as a high-income country by the World Bank standards. AB also has a high human development index which compares health, education and standard of living.[6]
Like other SIDS, AB is highly susceptible to climate change.[7] The terrain is flat with minimal annual rainfall, however global warming has increased extreme weather events including hurricanes and floods all of which make sustainable agriculture challenging.[7]
Historically, the first documented settlers in AB were the Arawaks, who introduced agriculture including the famous Antiguan black pineapple to the land.[8] However, the arrival of the Europeans in 1632, lead to the eradication of these indigenous people and massive importation of west African slaves to work the lands. The agricultural practices shifted to the monoculture of sugarcane production and propelled Antiguan people into an era of extreme poverty, malnutrition, and poor social health that lasted for centuries. In 1981, AB finally gained its independence and transitioned to a tourist-based economy which introduced the importation of new foods, and a vibrant growing economy.[8]

CHILDHOOD OBESITY IN ANTIGUA AND BARBUDA. Childhood obesity in AB has seen an exponential growth between 2000–2020.[9]

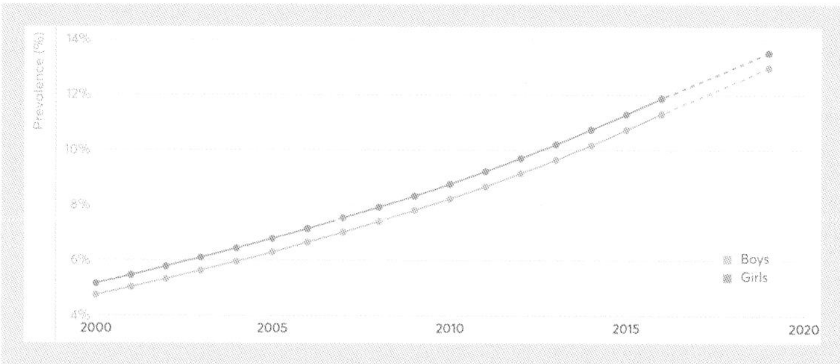

https://globalnutritionreport.org/resources/nutrition-profiles/latin-america-and-caribbean/caribbean/antigua-and-barbuda/ (last viewed December 2022)

Figure 1: Prevalence of obesity in children and adolescents in Antigua and Barbuda
Source: Global Nutrition Report Country Nutrition Profiles

Causes that have cultivated this obesogenic environment include physical inactivity, over-consumption of highly processed foods and sugar sweetened beverages (SSBs), insufficient access to water and fresh vegetables, socio-economic challenges, environmental challenges and the COVID 19 pandemic. Obesity does not discriminate as it impacts both high- and low-income countries and wealthy and impoverished persons.10 However, those living in poverty have poorer health outcomes. According to UNICEF in 2016, 25% of children and adolescents in AB were living in poverty, with a 6% higher incidence rate of poverty among female single-headed households.[11] Families have had to adapt to consuming more affordable processed & ultra-processed foods and SSBs with 70% of children consuming a soda per day.[12]

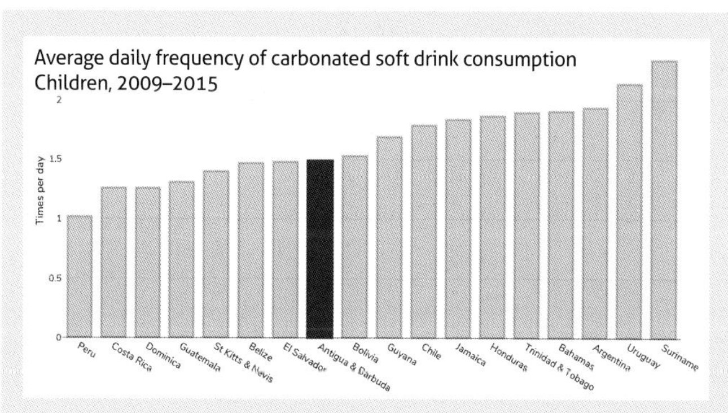

Figure 2: Average Daily Frequency of Carbonated Soft Drink Consumption

Source: Global Nutrition Report Country Nutrition Profiles https://globalnutritionreport.org/resources/nutrition-profiles/latin-america-and-caribbean/caribbean/antigua-and-barbuda/ (last viewed December 2022)

#02 Antigua
Combating Childhood Obesity in Antigua and Barbuda

In addition, increased utilization of public and private transportation, and the increased use of screens for recreation have decreased the participation of physical activity among children. Currently, physical activity in schools is only mandatory in government schools up to grade 9. Per week, children receive an average of 45 minutes of organized sport or play.[12] Combined with no access to bike lanes, limited sidewalks and suitable parks and recreations, children have limited opportunities to participate in physical activity.[13] Safety is another issue that increases physical inactivity among young girls. In 2016, 75% of male children ages 11–17 were inactive. In contrast, above 80% of female children 11–17 years of age were identified as physically inactive.[14]

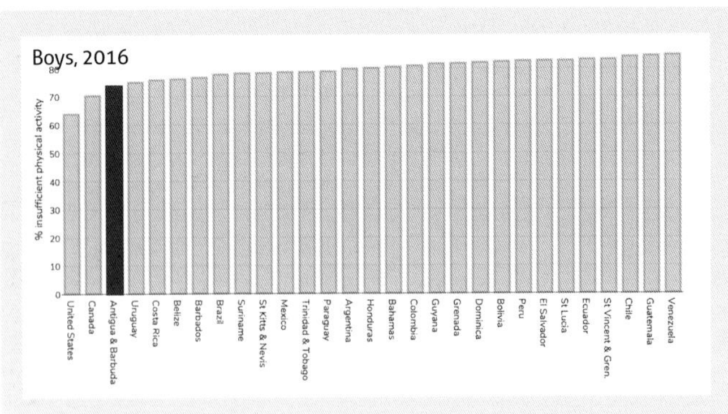

Figure 3: Insufficient physical activity, Boys Source: Report card: Antigua and Barbuda - data.worldobesity.org. (2022, October 28). Retrieved December 10, 2022, from https://data.worldobesity.org/country/antigua-and-barbuda-6/report-card.pdf

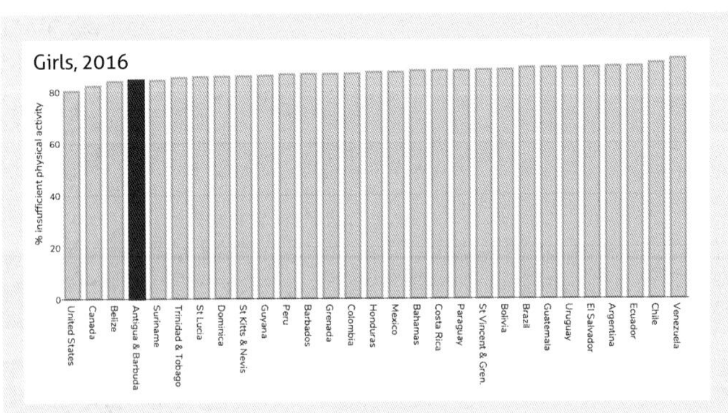

Figure 4: Insufficient physical activity, Girls Source: Report card: Antigua and Barbuda – data.worldobesity.org. (2022, October 28). Retrieved December 10, 2022, from https://data.worldobesity.org/country/antigua-and-barbuda-6/report-card.pdf

The impacts of the COVID 19 pandemic only exacerbated the issues related to poverty and physical inactivity thus fueling the childhood obesity crisis. Constant school closures, online learning and social distancing all decreased the already limited amount of physical activity children engaged in.[15] COVID 19 further increased the magnitude of poverty in AB with post pandemic estimations of children living in poverty increasing to from 25% to 29%.[11]

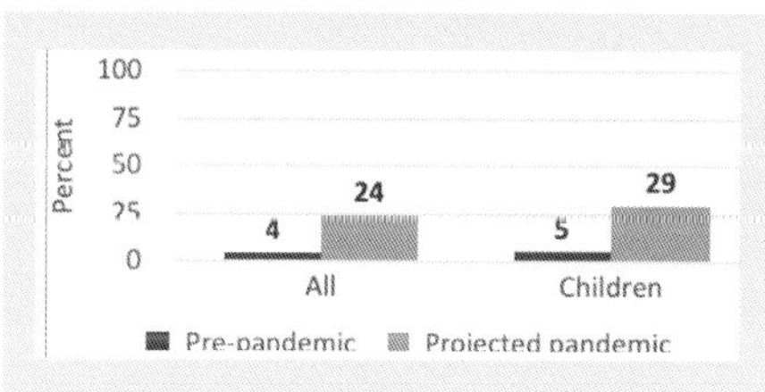

Figure 5: Projected changes in severe poverty due to COVID-19
Source: UNICEF Eastern Caribbean. UNICEF. (2021, July 1). Retrieved December 10, 2022, from https://www.unicef.org/easterncaribbean/

The leading reason for worsening poverty in AB was the impact of border closures on its tourist-based economy during COVID 19. This narrowed the fiscal space which led to budgetary cuts in the Medical Benefits Scheme (MBS), the country's health financing agency that finances health care for all residents through salary contributions.[16] During this time, community and school-based initiatives aimed at reducing childhood obesity were the first to be cut.

The growing economy in recent decades and the increased food insecurity of many households brought on by the pandemic fueled the obesogenic environment in AB. The health risks associated with obesity also severely impact the economy. The cost of obesity on health care was 6.5 million U.S dollars in 2016 and has been estimated to continue to increase reaching 125 million US dollars by 2025.[17]

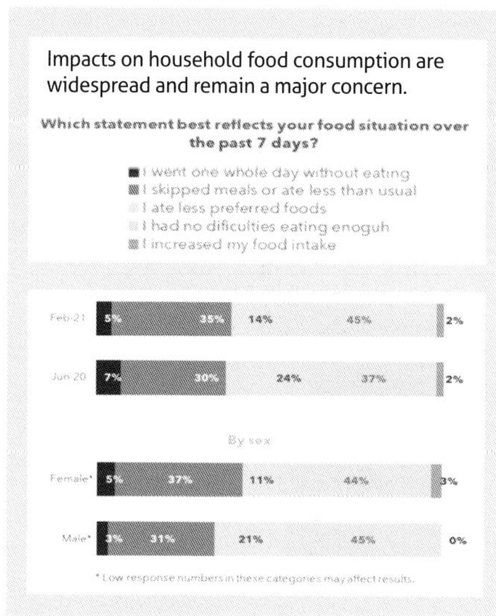

Figure 6: Prevalence of food consumption patterns in Antigua and Barbuda Households during the Covid 19 pandemic in June 2021
Source: Caribbean COVID-19 Food Security and Livelihoods Impact Survey Antigua and Barbuda Summary Report June 2021
https://docs.wfp.org/api/documents/WFP-0000129479/download/ last viewed December 2022

#02 Antigua
Combating Childhood Obesity in Antigua and Barbuda

METHODS. A literary review was conducted on reports addressing Obesity and Childhood Obesity from reputable sources including the United Nations (UN), WHO, PAHO, UNICEF, the World Obesity Federation, and the Global Nutrition Report. Additionally, the Nutrition Policy of Antigua and Barbuda, and other literature on nutrition and physical activity in AB were reviewed including the Healthy Caribbean Coalition report on Childhood Obesity. Finally, interviews were held with key stakeholders in AB in the Ministries of Health, Agriculture, Education and in the field of Public Health both locally and regionally.

DISCUSSION. CURRENT INTERVENTIONS & PROPOSED SOLUTION. AB has taken steps to reduce the prevalence and impact of obesity in the country. At the neonatal level, AB has multiple initiatives to increase exclusive breastfeeding among young mothers. This is crucial as optimal breastfeeding is linked to reduced risk of obesity and NCDs during childhood and in later life. Although, the Caribbean region as a whole holds one of the highest global breast-feeding averages, the regional average still falls below the global target of the WHO's Comprehensive Implementation Plan on Maternal, Infant and Young Child Nutrition to have at least 50% of all babies exclusively breastfed during the first six months of life by 2025.[18] To increase the exclusivity of breastfeeding, the country has initiated a National Breastfeeding Committee that has implemented a plethora of policies and programs to improve breast feeding practices.

For school aged children and beyond, there is a drafted policy awaiting implementation to enforce taxation on SSBs.[9] Taxing SSBs has been a great success in the neighboring country of Barbados, which after implementation in 2015, saw a substantial reduction in the sales and consumption of SSBs.[20] Enactment of this policy in AB shows promise of significantly decreasing sales and consumption of SSBs as well.

To further empower the AB communities and reduce food and water insecurities, the government introduced a Backyard Garden program (BYG) in association with the Food and Agricultural Organization (FAO), the National School Meals Program, Lifelong Learning for Farmers (L3F) and the Water Energy Nexus project[21][22][23]. Additionally, to address the limited physical activity of the AB population, in 2020 the government launched a national initiative called Antigua Barbuda Moves in hopes to reduce the incidence of noncommunicable disease (NCDs) such as diabetes and obesity.[24] This outreach initiative was curtailed by COVID but hosted a successful national walk in July 2022.[24] Feasible and sustainable solutions for AB will take multi-sectoral investment from the government, the public and private healthcare systems, schools, businesses, and the wider communities being served. This can be done by effectively strategizing the utilization and magnitude of the resources already present. For starters, focusing on incentivizing preventative care measures via the MBS. For example, the introduction of a tiered membership status based on positive lifestyle practices such as annual check-ups, regular exercise, NCD screenings and optimal management of associated chronic disorders may reduce healthcare costs while promoting members of the MBS to a silver, gold, or platinum status.

Next, there must be an improvement in the current data collection, analysis, access, and usage. Currently, there are local surveillance programs that are focused on children under age 5 years, however the information has been underutilized and should be consistently expanded to target all children under the age of 18.[9] To improve data resources, key data collectors and analyzers must be identified. For example, to monitor the weights of children during the school year, schools can collaborate with the health authorities by tracking BMI percentiles. In addition, the MBS can create an electronic platform to collect and maintain biometric and disease prevalence data. This will centralize the data, provide a snapshot of the country's health statistics, and provide appropriate electronic access to the government, the community, leaders, and policy writers. In addition, creating data driven policies that can be monitored, evaluated, and adjusted will improve financial decision making and health outcomes.

On a community level, an amplification of the school and home garden programs will reach more lower income families. This is currently being done within the L3F program which focuses on linking human, social and financial capital while empowering youth and women through farming.[13] Unfortunately, these programs have seen greater success within the middle- and higher-income families rather than those in greater need.[9] Through consistently enhanced targeted marketing in schools and the establishment of a resource sharing network between schools for seeds, crops, and soil will enable more lower income families to benefit from the program.

Lastly, for the proposed solutions to be successful and sustainable, there must be proper communication, community investment and confidence in the established programs. To ensure this community buy-in, the government of AB will need to ensure timely budgetary allocations and distributions within the fiscal year. In addition, improved intercommunication between the governmental ministries, healthcare systems and the Antiguan and Barbudan people is quintessential. In 2007, the Caribbean Community also known as CARICOM, recommended an inter-ministerial committee that focused on NCDs and health.[25] The successful implementation of this unit in Jamaica, can be used as a foundational framework for AB's different sectors to unite rather than continuing to work in silos.[26]

CONCLUSION. Childhood obesity is posing a grave threat globally as it leads to poor health and significant economic burden in high and low -income countries. It is linked to heart disease, type II diabetes, cancers, and low self-esteem. Its impact on a young nation such as AB can be crippling. It will take a systematic approach of government investments in data improvement and implementation of evidence-based policies. The mindset of holistic wellness must be embraced by the people of AB so that prevention can be prioritized further in the healthcare delivery model rather than the current treatment-based system.—

REFERENCES

1 World Health Organization. (n.d.). Obesity. World Health Organization. Retrieved December 10, 2022, from https://www.who.int/health-topics/obesity#tab=tab_1 **2** 07, S., & 08, S. (2022, September 26). Antigua and Barbuda - country profile. Health in the Americas. Retrieved October 7, 2022, from https://hia.paho.org/en/countries-22/antigua-barbuda-country-profile **3** World Health Organization. (2021, July 9). Obesity and overweight. World Health Organization. Retrieved December 11, 2022, from https://www.who.int/news-room/fact-sheets/detail/obesity-and-overweight **4** Centers for Disease Control and Prevention. (2022, July 15). Consequences of obesity. Centers for Disease Control and Prevention. Retrieved December 10, 2022, from https://www.cdc.gov/obesity/basics/consequences.html **5** United Nations. (n.d.). List of SIDS .:. sustainable development knowledge platform. United Nations. Retrieved December 10, 2022, from https://sustainabledevelopment.un.org/topics/sids/list **6** Antigua and barbuda - undp.org. (n.d.). Retrieved December 10, 2022, from https://www.undp.org/sites/g/files/zskgke326/files/migration/latinamerica/UNDP-RBLAC-BriefingNote-HumanDevelopmentReportBB.pdf **7** Climates for travelers. information on the climates in the world to plan A trip. Climates to Travel - world climate guide. (n.d.). Retrieved October 7, 2022, from https://www.climatestotravel.com/ **8** Kiple, K. F., & Ornelas, K. C. (Eds.). (2000). The Cambridge World History of Food. Cambridge University Press (Vol. 1). Cambridge University Press. Retrieved December 11, 2022, from https://doi.org/10.1017/CHOL9780521402149. **9** Country Nutrition Profiles. Global Nutrition Report | Country Nutrition Profiles - Global Nutrition Report. (n.d.). Retrieved October 7, 2022, from https://globalnutritionreport.org/resources/nutrition-profiles/latin-america-and-caribbean/caribbean/antigua-and-barbuda/ **10** A Food and Nutrition Security Policy for Antigua and Barbuda. Antigua and Barbuda Food and Nutrition Security Policy . (2012, September). Retrieved December 10, 2022, from https://extranet.who.int/nutrition/gina/sites/default/filesstore/ATG%202012%20FoodNutritionSecurityPolicyAG.pdf **11** UNICEF Eastern Caribbean. UNICEF. (2021, July 1). Retrieved December 10, 2022, from https://www.unicef.org/easterncaribbean/ **12** Jennelsa.Johnson. (2022, March 2). Childhood obesity: A problem that only gets worse as we fail to address it. Antigua Observer Newspaper. Retrieved October 7, 2022, from https://antiguaobserver.com/childhood-obesity-a-problem-that-only-gets-worse-as-we-fail-to-address-it/ **13** Walwyn, Danielle., & Walwyn , Dr. Leslie. (2022, September 13). Interview for GHT Caribbean Annual Conference . personal. **14** Report card: Antigua and barbuda - data.worldobesity.org. (2022, October 28). Retrieved December 10, 2022, from https://data.worldobesity.org/country/antigua and barbuda-6/report-card.pdf **15** Jennelsa.Johnson. (2022, March 2). Childhood obesity: A problem that only gets worse as we fail to address it. Antigua Observer Newspaper. Retrieved October 7, 2022, from https://antiguaobserver.com/childhood-obesity-a-problem-that-only-gets-worse-as-we-fail-to-address-it/ **16** 2021 budget statement - Antigua and Barbuda. (2022, February 3). Retrieved December 11, 2022, from https://ab.gov.ag/pdf/budget/Budget_Speech_2021.

pdf **17** Mitchell, C. (2017, January 18). Paho/WHO: Overweight affects almost half the population of all countries in Latin America and the Caribbean except for Haiti. Pan American Health Organization / World Health Organization. Retrieved October 7, 2022, from https://www3.paho.org/hq/index.php?option=com_content&view=article&id=12911%3Aoverweight-affects-half-population-latin-americacaribbean-except-haiti&Itemid=1926&lang=en#gsc.tab=0 **18** Hcc, & Hcc. (2021, August 12). The future talks: Infant and Young Child Nutrition - the first form of food security. Healthy Caribbean Coalition. Retrieved December 10, 2022, from https://www.healthycaribbean.org/the-future-talks-infant-and-young-child-nutrition-the-first-form-of-food-security/ **19** Walwyn, Dr.Leslie , & James, Juanita. (2022, September 5). Interview for GHT Caribbean Annual Conference . personal. **20** Alvarado, M., Unwin, N., Sharp, S. J., Hambleton, I., Murphy, M. M., Samuels, T. A., Suhrcke, M., & Adams, J. (2019, January 30). Assessing the impact of the Barbados sugar-sweetened beverage tax on beverage sales: An observational study - international journal of behavioral nutrition and physical activity. BioMed Central. Retrieved October 7, 2022, from https://ijbnpa.biomedcentral.com/articles/10.1186/s12966-019-0776-7 **21** Sidaner, E., Balaban, D., & Burlandy, L. (2012, December 6). The Brazilian School Feeding Programme: An example of an integrated programme in support of Food and Nutrition Security: Public Health Nutrition. Cambridge Core. Retrieved October 7, 2022, from https://www.cambridge.org/core/journals/public-health-nutrition/article/brazilian-school-feeding-programme-an-example-of-an-integrated-programme-in-s **22** Antigua and Barbuda to adopt l3f model. Commonwealth of Learning. (n.d.). Retrieved October 7, 2022, from https://www.col.org/news/antigua-and-barbuda-to-adopt-l3f-model/ **23** Fao – Water Energy Food Nexus Project. Ministry of Agriculture Fisheries and Barbuda Affairs FAO WATER ENERGY FOOD NEXUS PROJECT Comments. (n.d.). Retrieved December 10, 2022, from https://agriculture.gov.ag/index.php/2022/09/28/fao-water-energy-food-nexus-project/ **24** Team, M. (2022, May 30). Antigua Barbuda moves. Medical Benefits Scheme. Retrieved December 10, 2022, from https://www.mbs.gov.ag/v2/antigua-barbuda-moves/ **13** Antigua and Barbuda to adopt l3f model. Commonwealth of Learning. (n.d.). Retrieved October 7, 2022, from https://www.col.org/news/antigua-and-barbuda-to-adopt-l3f-model/ **25** Samuels, T. A., & Unwin, N. (2018, December 17). The 2007 Caribbean Community port-of-spain declaration on non-communicable diseases: An overview of a multidisciplinary evaluation. Revista panamericana de salud publica = Pan American journal of public health. Retrieved December 10, 2022, from https://www.ncbi.nlm.nih.gov/pmc/articles/PMC6385896/ **26** McIntosh, W. by: D. (2015, February 1). Inter-ministerial Committee to Oversee Poverty Alleviation Programmes. Jamaica Information Service. Retrieved December 10, 2022, from https://jis.gov.jm/inter-ministerial-committee-oversee-poverty-alleviation-programmes/

AUTHORS

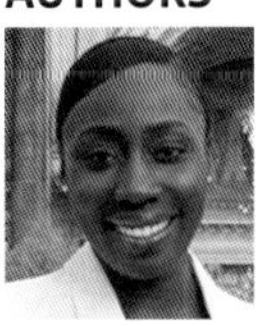

Nana Konadu-Asare MPH
Second year medical student, Global Health Track,
American University of Antigua College of Medicine

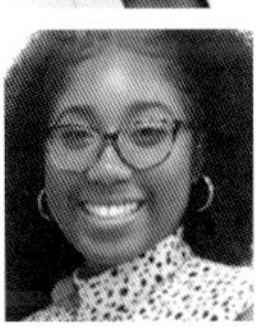

Ashleigh Bates
Second year medical student, Global Health Track,
American University of Antigua College of Medicine

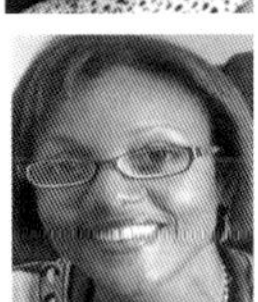

Leslie Walwyn MBBS, MPH
Professor Department of Clinical Medicine;
Associate Dean Global Health, American University of Antigua College of Medicine

#03 Gambia
Period Poverty: a global health issue affecting women and girls in The Gambia
Fatoumatta L. Kassama

ABOUT THE GAMBIA. The Gambia is the smallest country in mainland Africa, with an extent of about 330 km east to west, and less than 50 km north to south. The Gambia is one of the most densely populated countries in West Africa with a population of about 2.3 million people. The highest concentration of people is around the increasingly urbanized landscape spreading outward from The Gambia's capital, Banjul. The city is built on a small peninsula tucked between mangrove-lined estuaries and the broad mouth of the Gambia River, which rises out of the Fouta Djallon Highlands of Guinea. With its natural port, Banjul is an important trading post between West Africa and the world. The main ethnic groups are the Mandinka, the Wolof, and the Fula. The economy is largely based on agriculture and tourism, but it faces challenges such as high unemployment and poverty (Landscapes of West Africa, 2023).

CHALLENGES. More than 800 million people menstruate daily (Michel et al. 2022). Whereas 500 million lack access to menstrual products and adequate facilities (World Bank, 2023). Period poverty is a global health issue. It is a situation where menstruators lack access to adequate and hygienic sanitary products. They also lack knowledge of healthy period management practices and water, hygiene, and sanitation facilities to manage their period with dignity (World Bank, 2023). According to the study conducted by the Ministry of Basic and Secondary Education of The Gambia in 2018, girls miss 10-20% of school days in a year due to period poverty. When girls are absent from school, they miss a lot of lessons, perform poorly in class, and eventually drop out of school. When girls from low-income families drop out of school, they become victims of early or forced marriages, teenage pregnancies, and female genital mutilation (ActionAid, 2022). Some women and girls go through sexual violence or rape, domestic violence, emotional violence, or psychological violence in their communities in the process of accessing sanitary products. Less privileged women and girls resort to transactional sex. Transactional sex refers to non-commercial, non-marital sexual relationships where women and girls exchange sex for money so that they can buy sanitary products to manage their periods with dignity. This predisposes them to urogenital infections, STIs, HIV & AIDS, Herpes, and Cervical cancer. Recurrent urogenital infections can lead to infertility and thus cause physical or psychological violence in a girl's life. Period poverty results in mental health issues such as anxiety, depression, low self-esteem, suicidal thoughts, and suicide (Cardoso LF et al. 2021). Currently, girls and women especially those in rural Gambia use different unhygienic products to manage their periods. Some of the products include old pieces of cloth, rags, sponges, gauze, and toilet rolls. Those who use disposable pads do not dispose of them appropriately (ActionAid, 2022). On average, a menstruating person uses and disposes of 12,000 to 16,800 disposable sanitary products in their lifetime which is about 32 products each period (WoMena, 2019). Single-use menstrual products are made up of up to 90% plastic, and a cocktail of chemicals. Over a billion of these non-compostable sanitary products are making their way into sewerage systems, waterways, landfills, and water bodies every month causing harm to our environment, marine life, and human beings (Elledge et al. 2018). And every used sanitary napkin carries two grams of non-biodegradable plastic (WEN, 2018). The amount of non-biodegradable plastic accumulated every month is very high, a factor strong enough to raise concern over the crisis which the environment is facing currently. It is estimated that 1 disposable pad is equivalent to 4 plastic bags and if buried, it can spend 500-800 years in the ground (Friend of the Earth, 2018). The issue of managing menstrual waste needs more attention, however, it is the most neglected topic in the menstrual health and hygiene management value chain, water sanitation and hygiene, and climate change.

ABOUT GIRLS PRIDE. Girls' Pride Gambia is a non-profit, women-led, community-based organization that started in 2017 as a result of period poverty affecting girls' education in The Gambia. It provides sustainable, eco-friendly, and reusable sanitary pads for women and girls from low-income families, trains women, men, and adolescent boys and girls on sexual and reproductive health and rights (SRHR) through gamification, conducts training of trainers on SRHR, training on reusable sanitary pad production, and offers online and offline counselling services. Girls' Pride Gambia's mission is to create an inclusive safe space and promote the utilization of sustainable solutions for sexual and reproductive health and well-being for all and its vision is to provide access to comprehensive health education and healthy sexual and reproductive health products and services through innovation. Girls' Pride Gambia is working on different objectives to address sexual and reproductive health issues and advance gender equality in The Gambia. Some of their objectives include:

- To keep girls in schools during their periods through the provision of menstrual health and hygiene management education and the distribution of reusable, eco-friendly, and biodegradable sanitary pads.
- End sexual and gender-based violence and harmful traditional practices such as female genital mutilation and child marriage.

#03 Gambia
Period Poverty: a global health issue affecting women and girls in The Gambia

- End inequalities by involving women and girls from low-income and underserved communities, persons with disabilities, displaced individuals, refugees, prisoners, and orphans.
- End gender inequality by empowering adolescent boys and girls, men, and women on sexual and reproductive health and rights.
- Eradicate the stigma, social norms and taboos surrounding sexual and reproductive health and rights, gender-based violence and harmful traditional practices in The Gambia.
- Reduce the amount of plastic waste generated during menstruation from single-used disposable pads and tampons that are causing harm to the environment and waterbodies through the provision of environmentally friendly and reusable sanitary pads that generate zero waste and reduce the carbon footprints of menstruators.
- Conduct skills training for women and girls on how to make reusable sanitary pads using biodegradable materials that are locally available in their communities.
- Girls' Pride Gambia recruits women and girls from low-income families, divorcees, and survivors of sexual and gender-based violence, child marriage, and female genital mutilation as community volunteers and empowers them with the right knowledge and skills they need to become advocates in their local communities.

Through their various community projects, Girls' Pride Gambia is advancing the following UN Sustainable Development Goals (SDGs).

- ***SDG 3 – Good Health and Wellbeing***
- ***SDG 4 – Quality Education***
- ***SDG 5 – Gender Quality***
- ***SDG 6 – Clean Water and Sanitation***
- ***SDG 8 – Decent job and economic growth***
- ***SDG 10 – Reduce inequalities.***
- ***SDG 12 – Responsible consumption and production***
- ***SDG 13 – Climate Change***

HOW GIRLS' PRIDE IS ADDRESSING PERIOD POVERTY IN THE GAMBIA. Girls' Pride Gambia works with its partners and community volunteers to raise awareness about sexual and reproductive health and rights, harmful traditional practices, sexual and gender-based violence, how they can eradicate the negative social norms, and taboos in The Gambia and the impact of climate change on human health. The NGO provides healthy,environmentally friendly, and reusable sanitary pads for women and girls from low-income families, marginalized communities, persons with disabilities, internally displaced women and girls, orphans, prisoners, and girls who live in boarding schools. To sustain their projects, they involve community members to take ownership of the projects and provide the little resources that are locally available in their communities. Some of the projects they have implemented with their partners include:

Project Thrive is an initiative that trains vulnerable women and girls on menstrual hygiene management and provides eco-friendly and reusable sanitary pads for them to thrive in their communities. They conduct school and community sensitization programs for girls on menstrual hygiene, period shaming, harmful traditional practices, and sexual and gender-based violence. Girls' Pride Gambia works with celebrities and models during miss competitions and fashion shows and uses those platforms to educate people about period poverty and how it affects girls' education. They also conduct training of trainer programs on reusable sanitary pad production. Through their partnership with the Comprehensive Health Education Project under the Ministry of Basic and Secondary Education (MoBSE), twenty-six (26) schoolteachers were trained on how to make handmade reusable sanitary pads. Each of these teachers set up reusable pad banks in their schools and also continues training their students- both boys and girls on how to make sanitary pads. Boys make pads for their schoolmates and girls make pads for themselves. Some of the reusable pads are kept in the pad banks in schools. The pad bank is a safe corner in schools where girls get access to reusable and eco-friendly sanitary pads during their periods. Girls' Pride Gambia believes that they cannot achieve gender equality without men and boys. Therefore, they train men and adolescent boys on sexual and reproductive health and rights. They empower men and boys to become advocates for women's and girls' rights in their local communities and to understand that women and girls can make decisions about their bodies on their own.

In May 2022, they launched the #Tree-4Pads project. This is a community climate change mitigation project that involves adolescent girls and young women in tree-planting exercises. They partner with organizations that work on climate change and nature conservation. Women and girls are educated on climate change, the impact of climate change on their health and how using reusable and environmentally friendly sanitary products can reduce their carbon footprints and allow them to manage their periods with dignity. For each tree planted, girls and young women receive sanitary pads that are reusable for 3 years.

Currently, Girls' Pride Gambia uses gamification- the Funneh board game to educate adolescent girls, boys and adults about global health and planetary health issues such as menstruation, teenage pregnancy, child marriage, female genital mutilation, mental health, contraceptives, HIV& AIDS, and climate change. Introducing their community

#03 Gambia
Period Poverty: a global health issue affecting women and girls in The Gambia

members to learning through gamification gives them the opportunity to initiate and normalize conversations around complex, sensitive and taboo topics in schools, at home and in workplaces.

In July 2022, Girls' Pride Gambia partnered with eTrash2Cash on a project called #Plastics4Pads. Through this project, women and girls have the opportunity to exchange household plastic waste with reusable and eco-friendly sanitary pads. The plastic waste that is collected is sent to recycling companies that recycle plastic waste to reduce the number of plastics in their environment and protect the water bodies from plastic pollution. Girls' Pride Gambia's volunteers also train adolescent girls in rural communities on how to repurpose some of the plastic waste into useful household materials.

The non-profit community-based organization Girls' Pride Gambia has thirty-five (35) team members and over fifteen (15) local and international partners. They have distributed over 15,000 eco-friendly and reusable sanitary pads, and over 20,000 people were educated on issues related to sexual and reproductive health and rights and climate change. Seven-six (76) people including schoolteachers and community members were trained on how to make reusable sanitary pads. One hundred and sixty (160) schoolteachers from conventional and non-conventional schools were trained on menstrual hygiene management, gender-based violence, and period shaming and the majority of the teachers trained were male teachers. With support from media houses in The Gambia, Girls' Pride Gambia has conducted about 50 TV and community radio sensitization programs to educate Gambians on sexual and reproductive health, and rights and how they can work together to address the taboos in their communities. Through the #Tree4Pads initiative, over 3000 trees have been planted in our communities to restore the ecosystem.—

REFERENCES

1 ActionAid (May 2022). Period poverty: the statistics around the world. Retrieved from https://www.actionaid.org.uk/blog/2022/05/18/period-poverty-statistics-around-world **2** Cardoso LF, Scolese AM, Hamidaddin A, Gupta J. Period poverty and mental health implications among college-aged women in the United States. BMC Women's Health. 2021;21(1):14. doi:10.1186/s12905-020-01149-5 **3** Elledge, M., Muralidharan, A., Parker, A., Ravndal, K., Siddiqui, M., Toolaram, A. and Woodward, K., 2018. Menstrual Hygiene Management and Waste Disposal in Low and Middle Income Countries—A Review of the Literature. International Journal of Environmental Research and Public Health, 15(11), p.2562. **4** Friends of the Earth(2018). Plastic periods: menstrual products and plastic pollution. Retrieved from https://friendsoftheearth.uk/sustainable-living/plastic-periods-menstrual-products-and-plastic-pollution **5** Landscapes of West Africa: a window on a changing world (2023, February 4th). The Republic of The Gambia. Retrieved from https://eros.usgs.gov/westafrica/country/republic-gambia **6** Michel J, Mettler A, Schönenberger S, Gunz D. Period poverty: why it should be everybody's business. Journal of Global Health Reports. 2022;6:e2022009. doi:10.29392/001c.32436 **7** Ministry of Basic and Secondary Education 2018. The impact of the supply of sanitary pads on girls' education. Retrieved from http://www.edugambia.gm/advertistments/study-reveals-girls-lose-10-20-

school-days-during-menstruation. **8** World Bank (2023, February 3rd). Menstrual Health and Hygiene. Retrieved from https://www.worldbank.org/en/topic/water/brief/menstrual-health-and-hygiene **9** Women's Environmental Network (WEN). WEN Stat On usage. 2018. Retrived from: https://www.london.gov.uk/sites/default/files/plastics_unflushables_-_submited_evidence.pdf **10** WoMena 2019. What is the Environmental Impact of Menstrual Products? Retrieved from https://womena.dk/what-is-the-environmental-impact-of-menstrual-products/

AUTHOR

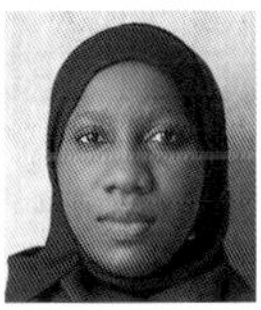

Fatoumatta L. Kassama (Founder & CEO)
Girls' Pride Gambia | Banjul, The Gambia, West Africa
Fellow International Sustainability Academy 2022
Tel: (+220) 9991280/2627516 | E-mail: girlspridegambia@gmail.com
FACEBOOK: https://www.facebook.com/girlspridegambia
TWITTER: https://twitter.com/GirlsPrideGam?s=03
INSTAGRAM: https://www.instagram.com/girlspridegambia/?hl=en

GIRLS' PRIDE

institute for
RESEARCH IN
INTERNATIONAL ASSISTANCE

IRIA – INTERNATIONAL ACTIVITIES 03.2023

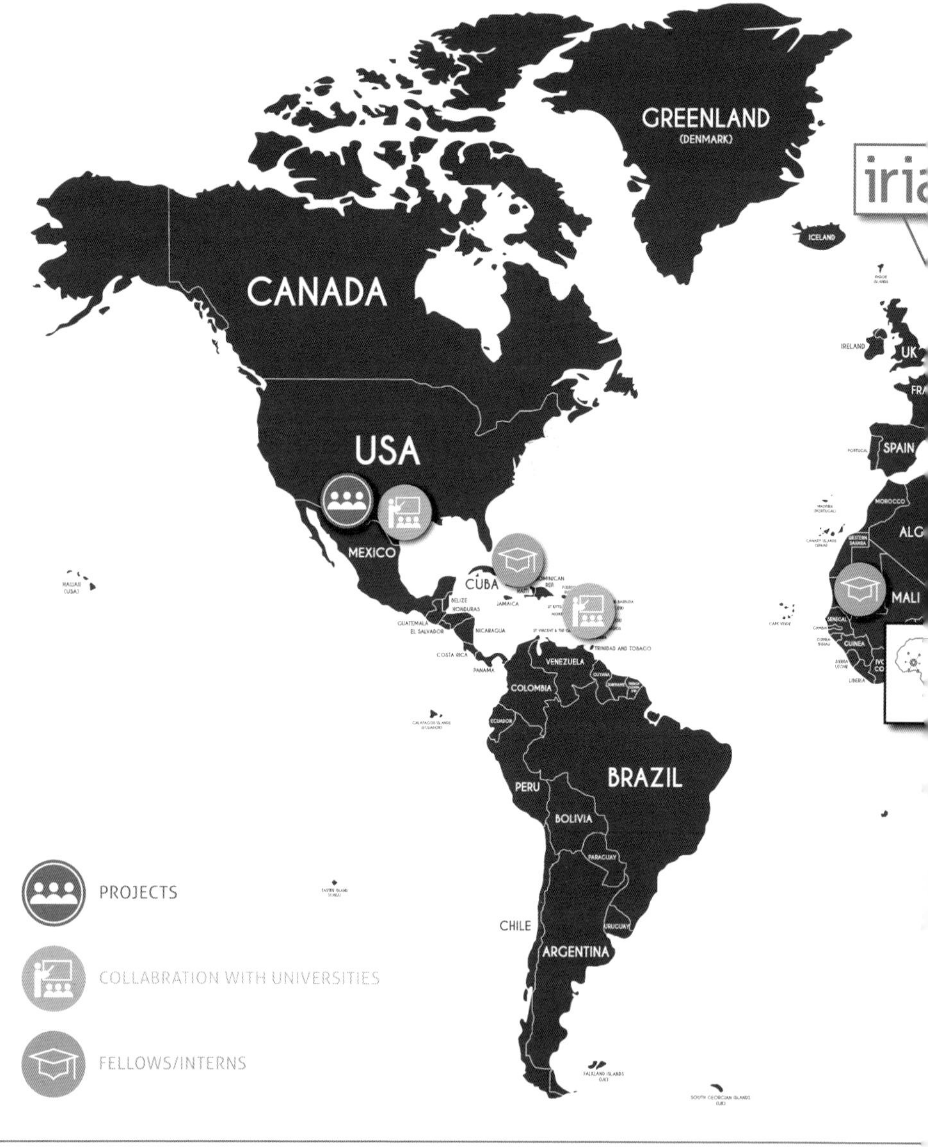

akkon
HOCHSCHULE FÜR
HUMANWISSENSCHAFTEN

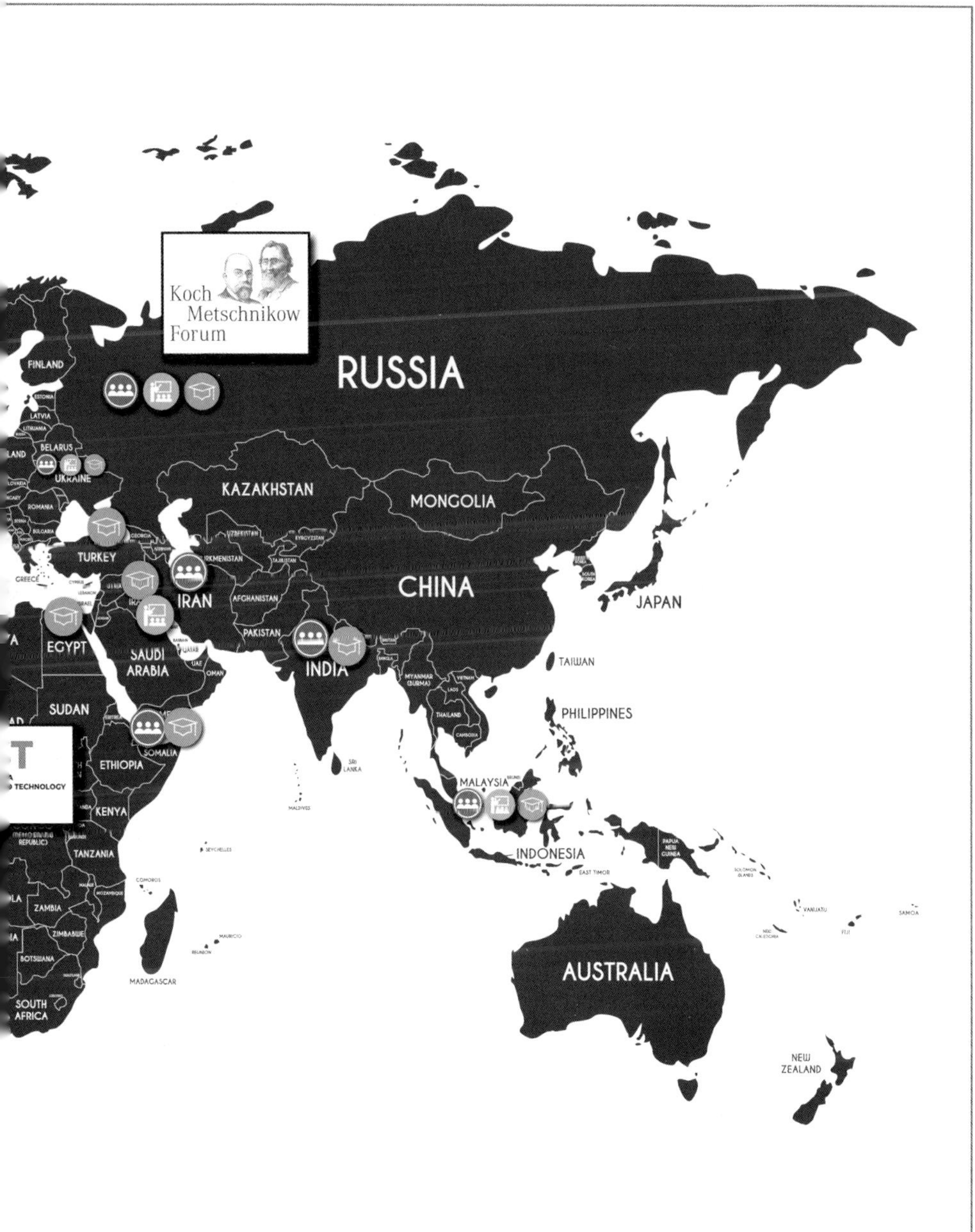

#04.1 Ghana
Spatial Epidemiology of Bacterial Meningitis in the Upper West Region of Ghana: The Effect of Climate Change on the Disease Burden

Ali Musah, Asori Moses, Emmanuel K. Nakua

ABSTRACT. BACKGROUND. The use of GIS has been crucial in modeling disease risk for rapid and effective surveillance. Particularly, it has been used by researchers to evaluate environmental factors associated with meningitis risk. Despite these advantages, its use has been extremely limited in the Upper West Region of Ghana. This study used GIS and spatial statistics to model spatially varying predictors of meningitis prevalence.

METHODS. Health data were collected between 2018 and 2020, to examine spatiotemporal associations. All cases were geocoded at the community level. Spatial modeling was done with Geographic Weighted Regression (GWR) model to determine the spatial variation in the relationship between meningitis incidence and bioclimatic conditions.

RESULTS. Between 2018 and 2022, a total of 1,176 cases of bacterial meningitis were reported, resulting in 118 fatalities. Of these cases, 605 were male and 571 were female, with the age group of 15-29 years being the most affected. The highest Attack Rate (AR) was observed in Nandom at 492 per 100,000 population, followed by Nadowli-Kaleo at 314 per 100,000 population. Conversely, Jirapa had the highest Case Fatality Rate (CFR) at 17%. The GWR model analysis revealed that precipitation (r2=0.93), wind speed (r2=0.8), and household size (r2=0.56) were positively associated with the prevalence of bacterial meningitis.

CONCLUSION. Household size and windspeed place a significant role in the spread of meningitis. Therefore, time and targeted interventions should be directed toward areas and communities with larger household sizes and higher average windspeed.

KEYWORDS. Spatial Epidemiology, Bioclimatic Conditions, Climate Change, Bacterial Meningitis, Geospatial Analysis, Ghana, and Upper West Region

INTRODUCTION. Meningitis is a health condition characterized by inflammation of the meninges, the protective membranes surrounding the brain and spinal cord, and/or the cerebrospinal fluid (Joseph et al., 2020; WHO, 2011b). It can be caused by various pathogenic agents, including viruses, fungi, and bacteria (AM & MC Thomson, 2002; Putz et al., 2013). However, the majority of meningitis cases are caused by bacteria, particularly Neisseria meningitidis (serogroups A, W135, C, and X), Streptococcus pneumoniae (S.P), and Haemophilus influenzae type B (Hib). Meningitis outbreaks are associated with social, economic, and healthcare burdens in low-income settings due to the frequency of outbreaks (Souza et al., 2012). Transmission of meningitis is frequently associated with fluid secretion from the throat and the transfer of infected droplets to an infected person (Paireau et al., 2012). Meningitis can cause permanent brain damage and other permanent sequelae, and evidence shows that if left untreated, meningitis can cause serious brain injury in 15% of cases (WHO, 2018, 2021). While meningitis can occur anywhere at any time, people in Sub-Saharan Africa (SSA) are at greater risk (Edward, 2020). The meningitis belt, a region in SSA stretching from Senegal to Ethiopia, experiences annual outbreaks, which occur during the dry season between October and May, characterized by dryness and dust (Paireau et al., 2012). Historically, these yearly outbreaks have been associated with Neisseria meningitidis serogroup A (NmA) (AJ Pollard, 2004). Globally, there are more than 1.2 million cases of bacterial meningitis every year (WHO, 1997). Without timely intervention, case fatality may reach 70%, and at least 20% of cases are likely to have permanent sequelae, such as hearing loss, limb amputation, and neurological disability (WHO, 2011a). However, the prevalence and mortality of meningitis vary according to sociodemographics, geography, and prevailing bioclimatic conditions (CDC, 2016). The Northern, North East, Savanna, Upper East, and West, and the Bono East Regions are at greater risk of bacterial meningitis since they are located within the meningitis belt (Hodgson et al., 2001), and most NnA epidemics have historically occurred in these regions. For example, between 1996 and 1997, there was a large-scale outbreak where 18,703 cases and 1356 deaths were recorded, and all these cases occurred within districts within the three northern regions (Tikhomirova et al., 1997). There was a combined outbreak of S. Pneumoniae and Neisseria Meningitidis Serotype W (NmW) between 2015 and 2016 that affected the entire Ghana, even though Upper West and Brong Ahafo Regions were the most affected in the country (Aku et al., 2017; Domo et al., 2017; Kwarteng et al., 2017a). There have also been focal outbreaks in these regions caused by serotype NmW since 2010 (Kwarteng et al., 2017b; Kwarteng et al., 2017a). However, there has been a significant decline in cases caused by Neisseria Meningitidis Serotype A (NmA) since the introduction of Polysaccharide Conjugate Vaccine Type A during the early 2000s (Carod Artal, 2015; Ferraro et al., 2014). The outbreaks in Upper West in particular have been experiencing seasonal outbreaks usually between October and April every year.

#04.1 Ghana
Spatial Epidemiology of Bacterial Meningitis in the Upper West Region of Ghana: The Effect of Climate Change on the Disease Burden

Since all districts within the district are situated within the meningitis belt and are all affected by the dry season (Harmattan), there is a significant disease burden. For example, the cooccurrence of Neisseria Meningitidis serotype X (NmX) and Covid-19 outbreaks in 2020 posed a serious health burden to the public health system in the region (Ali et al., 2022a; GHS, 2020). Despite the demonstrable burden, management of the epidemics remains very difficult in Ghana particularly in Upper West, partly due to the spatiality of the occurrence. Due to the spatiality of the epidemics, without effective and targetable intervention such as surveillance, it may be difficult to optimize scarce resources. Considering the seasonality of the epidemics, it may be logical to argue they may be an association between certain bioclimatic factors and bacterial meningitis. There is also a challenge of improving surveillance efforts due to spatial sociodemographic heterogeneity. For example, household size may vary significantly across the region. Considering the fuzzy nature of bioclimatic conditions, it is difficult to describe its influence on epidemics descriptively. Since risk factor(s) guided information may be useful to targetable intervention, and the fact that some of these risk factors spatially vary, there is the need to design models that estimate spatially varying relationships. However, currently, there is no study focusing on the spatial epidemiology of bacterial meningitis based on bioclimatic drivers. This research gap poses a significant challenge to effective management and prevention efforts. This study, therefore, adopts geographically weighted regression (GWR) to geographically varying relationships between meningitis prevalence and annual precipitation, wind speed, and household size.

MATERIALS AND METHODS

Study Area

Upper West Region is found in the North Western flank of Ghana covering a land area of 18,476 km2. It is bordered to the north and west by Burkina Faso, east by Upper East Region, and South by Brong Regions. It has a population of approximately 901,499 people in 2022, calculated using a 2.0% rate of growth from the Population and Housing Census 2020 (GSS, 2020). Bio-climatically, the region is predominantly a guinea savanna with a topical climate. It has a minimum temperature of 22.60C and a maximum of 40.10C, and precipitation of between 100 and 120cm per year. Harmattan winds during the dry season are characterized by dust originating from the Sahara, in the Northeastern part of the region. This period is known for colder nights and dry/dusty daytime. The combination of these climatic conditions makes the region extremely vulnerable to seasonal meningitis outbreaks (GHS, 2020).

Study Design

This was a retrospective spatial epidemiologic study design where retrospective data between 2018 and 2020 were considered. This data was collected through routine surveillance in the Upper West Region.

Study Population

All cases were included independent of age or sex or any sociodemographic factors. However, cases that did not meet the WHO standard case definition (suspected, probable, and confirmed cases) of bacterial meningitis were excluded. The case definitions used for this criterion were:

1. Suspected Meningitis Case: Any person with abrupt onset of fever (>38.5 °C), neck stiffness, or other meningeal signs, including bulging fontanelle in infants, was considered a suspected case. (IDSR-GHS, 2019)

2. Probable Meningitis Case: Suspect a case with turbid, cloudy, or purulent appearance of cerebrospinal fluid (CSF) sample or leukocyte count >10 cells/mm3 or with bacteria identified by Gram stain in CSF, or positive antigen detection in CSF. (IDSR-GHS, 2019)

3. Confirmed Meningitis Case. Cases that were identified by laboratory confirmation by bacteria culture, Polymerase Chain Reaction (PCR) (test for the identification of Neisseria Meningitidis, Streptococcus Pneumonia, Haemophilus influenza type B) in CSF or blood were considered the confirmed case. (IDSR-GHS, 2019)

Defining the Study Variables

Key data elements extracted include the epidemiological week, name of sub-district, name of the district, the community of origin, geographical location of the cases (GPS coordinates), sex, date first seen at the health facility, signs, and symptoms (fever, neck stiffness, headache), outcome, date of onset signs & symptoms, vaccination status of the case, specimen collected, the date the specimen was collected, laboratory test results (Gram, TDR, Latex, Culture, PCR), and the final classification of cases.

DATA COLLECTION AND PROCESSING

Extraction of Meningitis and Household Data

Data were retrieved from the line list of meningitis cases from routine surveillance data with a data extraction sheet. Individual references were made on case-based forms and laboratory tests in case of missing data from the database. Exploration and checks for completeness were done to improve accuracy and reliability. The extraction exercise was carried out by the regional surveillance officer and the primary investigator, and any disagreement was resolved. Average household size data were also extracted from the quarterly Community-Based Health Planning and Services (CHPS) database for the years 2018–2020.

#04.1 Ghana
Spatial Epidemiology of Bacterial Meningitis in the Upper West Region of Ghana: The Effect of Climate Change on the Disease Burden

Spatial and Bio-Climatic Data

For spatial modeling, all cases were georeferenced with geographical coordinates that defined their spatial locations. Since there is no address locator for automated geocoding purposes, the geocoding exercise was done manually using Google Maps. Placemarks were specifically utilized to retrieve spatial information and converted to a feature class in the GIS environment. Geographic unit data (administrative level 1 and 2 boundaries) were extracted from the Ghana Health Service DHIMS-2 platform. To evaluate the bioclimatic impacts, we downloaded precipitation and windspeed data from WorldClim (https://www.worldclim.org/). Precipitation and windspeed were raster datasets and had to be pre-processed for vector-based spatial modeling. The downloaded data were projected using UTM Zone 30 N. Since the spatial resolution was 500m, we resampled to 100m using the bilinear resample technique. The re-projected data was clipped to our study area. We calculated the mean rainfall and windspeed for individual sub-districts using zonal statistics.

DATA ANALYSIS

Descriptive Statistics

Categorical variables were summarized as frequencies and percentages, while continuous variables were summarized as means. To describe temporal trends, we used an epidemiologic curve. The simple spatial distribution of the cases was mapped to discern the spatial pattern of occurrence, and incidences of bacterial meningitis were computed. The analysis was done using STATA and ArcGIS 10.5.

Assessing the Impact of Bio-Climatic Dynamic Influence on Meningitis Prevalence

For an efficient, effective, and economically sound way of tackling meningitis, surveillance and resource allocation should be spatially targeted. Bio-climatic factors were used as predictors to understand how these variables may predict the spatial pattern of the disease. The direction of influence of these imposed predictive variables was examined spatially. Classical regression models such as global ordinary least squares (OLS) are spatial and, thus, do not consider spatial heterogeneity (Mansour et al., 2020). It is assumed that all phenomena vary continuously across places, so residuals are considered purely unstructured. However, almost all geographic phenomena, including diseases such as meningitis and their driving factors, are spatial (van Donkelaar et al., 2018). Therefore, the classical regression model may fail to reveal the true association across space for targetable intervention. We, therefore, adopted geographically weighted regression (GWR). The GWR model is specified in Equation 1 as follows:

$$Yi = \beta 0\ (ui, vi) + \sum k\ \beta k\ (ui, vi)\ xik + \varepsilon i$$

Where (u_i, v_i) is the geographical coordinates of point i and $\beta_k (u_i, v_i)$ is the calculated coefficient of association in a particular geographical unit or location i. $\beta_0 (u_i, v_i)$ is the locational intercept of the model and ε_i is the error term associated with the model. GWR calibrates localized models across space using mathematically defined neighbors to evaluate how localized relationships may vary from one location to the other (Asori, Musah, & Peprah, 2022; van Donkelaar et al., 2018). We used variable bandwidths to define the neighborhood radius for meningitis cases. Even though multiple kernel functions exist for defining an optimal variable bandwidth, we adopted the Gaussian model, where the impact of neighbors on the central feature diminished but never reaches zero (Asori, Musah, & Gyasi, 2022). This was necessary to account for the fuzzy nature of spatial dependencies. As a result of this flexible model, the relationship between meningitis prevalence and bio-climatic variables such as rainfall and wind conditions was made to vary across space which reflects real-world phenomenal behavior.

Ethical Consideration

Ethical approval was obtained from the Kwame Nkrumah University of Science and Technology's (KNUST) Committee on Human Research, Publication, and Ethics (Ref Number: CHRPE/AP/270/21), and permission and approval were granted by the Ghana Health Service. All traceable identifiers associated with the cases were masked. GPS coordinates of the cases' locations were randomly dotted within the community of origin with subdistrict centroids, concealing the exact geographical locations of the households of the cases.

RESULTS

Descriptive Epidemiology

The data analysis involved 1,176 cases of bacterial meningitis recorded in the study area within three years between 2018 and 2020. It was observed that a total of 118 deaths and 1,058 survivors were recorded within the same period under study (Figure 1.0). Of all the bacterial meningitis cases recorded, 605 were males and 571 were females while the age group < 1 year was the least affected. Age groups 5-14 years and 15-29 were the most affected with 255 and 265 cases respectively.

It was also found that the incidence of meningitis within the three years studied followed a cyclical trend as shown in prompting the need to monitor these epidemiological weeks for timely intervention. The majority of the cases usually occur between epidemiological weeks 2 – 17 for all three years compared (2018, 2019, and 2020). These periods represent environmentally favorable conditions for the transmission of the epidemics such as the predominance of dust, low humidity, and increased wind

#04.1 Ghana
Spatial Epidemiology of Bacterial Meningitis in the Upper West Region of Ghana: The Effect of Climate Change on the Disease Burden

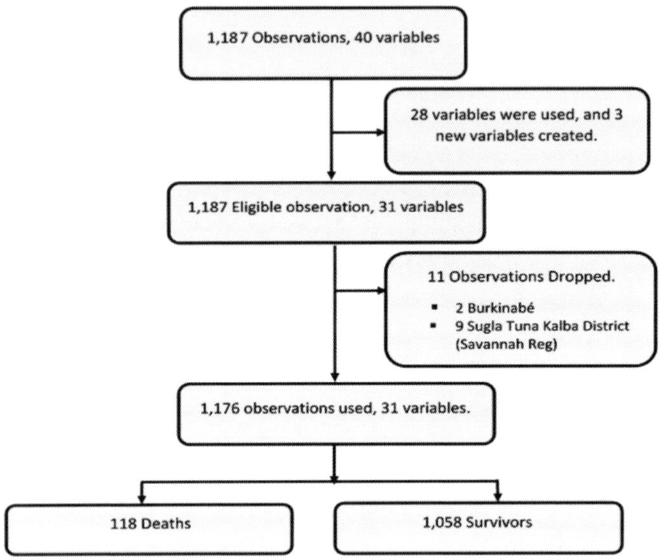

Figure 1.0 Data Structure and Variables | Source: Field Data

speed. For the three years, the prevalence of meningitis cases was 52 per 100,000 population, 41 per 100,000 population, and 48 per 100,000 population for 2018, 2019, and 2020 respectively. Comparatively, the 2020 Case Fatality Rate (CFR) was 13.6% which is almost two folds higher than 2019 (CFR 7.6%) and 2018 (CFR 9.0%). This is an indication that the temporal trajectory of the fatality is much gloomier in the future if no intervention mechanism is not devised.

Results also indicate that Nandom had the highest Attach Rate (AR) of 492 per 100,000 population, followed closely by Nadowli-Kaleo with an AR of 314 per 100,000 population as they recorded the highest attack rates. These observed cases of meningitis, however, do not depict a population-cases ratio, as Nandom has a population quite lower (55,925) than Nadowli (74,507) indicating a relatively, severe health burden in Nandom.

ASSESSING THE SPATIAL DISTRIBUTION OF MENINGITIS PREVALENCE

From Figure 2.0 below, it is apparent that the spatial distribution of the cases is not out of random chance, as homogeneity has not been observed. The north-western part of the region has more clusters than the eastern flank, as a sparing incidence of the disease was observed. This, therefore, warranted the investigation of spatial and temporal consistency in the observed distribution of the disease incidence. To implement this, the current study utilized a Spatio-temporal approach to examine the spatial trend of the incidence from 2018 to 2020 based on prevalence measures cases/100,000 population.

gion in 2018. These are urban centers and therefore population density and size were relatively higher. Therefore, a higher incidence was expected as discovered in some studies. In 2018, four very high prevalence clusters were observed. However, there was a gradual spatial diffusion of the prevalence towards the middle belt of the study area in 2019. This spatial growth continued in 2020 as the prevalence of meningitis

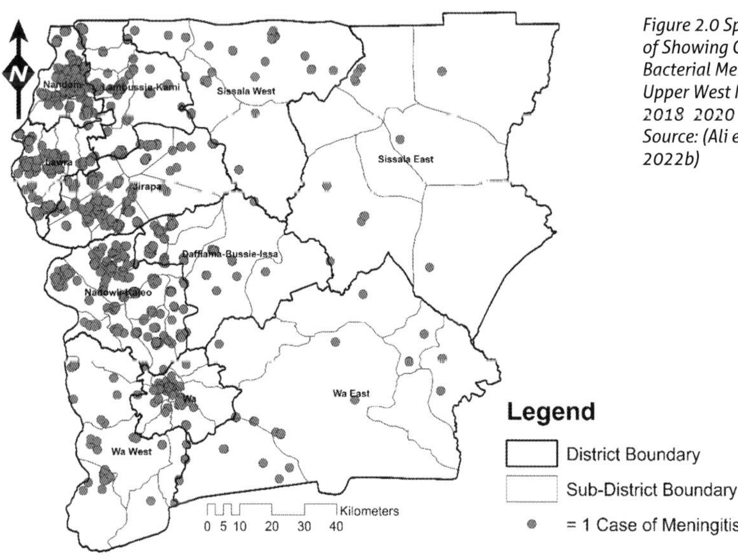

Figure 2.0 Spot Map of Showing Cases of Bacterial Meningitis, Upper West Region, 2018 2020 Source: (Ali et al., 2022b)

The result shows that the incidence of meningitis was high around the north-western and the Middle Western part (Nandom, Jirapa, Lawra, Lambussie, and Nadowli-Kaleo) of the Upper West Re-

was widespread from the west to many parts of the region. It is therefore apparent that the spatial growth or diffusion will continue in the near if intervention mechanisms are not devised.

#04.1 Ghana
Spatial Epidemiology of Bacterial Meningitis in the Upper West Region of Ghana: The Effect of Climate Change on the Disease Burden

IMPACT OF THE BIO-CLIMATIC CONDITION ON MENINGITIS PREVALENCE GEOGRAPHICALLY WEIGHTED REGRESSION (GWR). In exploring the reason behind spatial heterogeneity in the distribution of meningitis in the Upper West Region. It was found that the Geographically Weighted Regression (GWR) model better explained the relationship between meningitis incidence and rainfall (R2 = 0.93; AICCs = 510.87) as opposed to the Ordinary Least Squares (OLS) (R2 = 0.27; AICCs = 584.16). These results demonstrated that the association between meningitis prevalence and precipitation (rainfall) does not follow a homogenous spatial order but varies significantly in space.

Due to the impact of wind on the spread of droplets of diseases (Sultan et al., 2005a), This current study also investigated how wind speed aids in explaining the distribution of meningitis in the region. It was also found that, based on the GWR model, wind speed on the contrary had a stronger positive influence on meningitis cases (R2 = 0.80; AICCs = 668) than the OLS model (R2 = 0.07; AICCs = 601.72). Comparing Figure 2.0 and Figure 4.0 it is apparent that the association between meningitis and wind speed was stronger where the prevalence was also high and got spatially weaker towards the middle part of the region where people have sparingly settled.

Table 1.0 Comparison of Ordinary Least Square (OLS) and Geographic Weighted Regression (GWR) Models

Variables	OLS Model		GWR Model	
	AICc	R2	AICc	R2
Precipitation	584.61	0.27	510.87	0.93
Wind Speed	601.72	0.07	-363.62	0.80
Household Size	599.63	0.14	598.48	0.56

AICc = Aikaike Information criterion

Source: Field Data

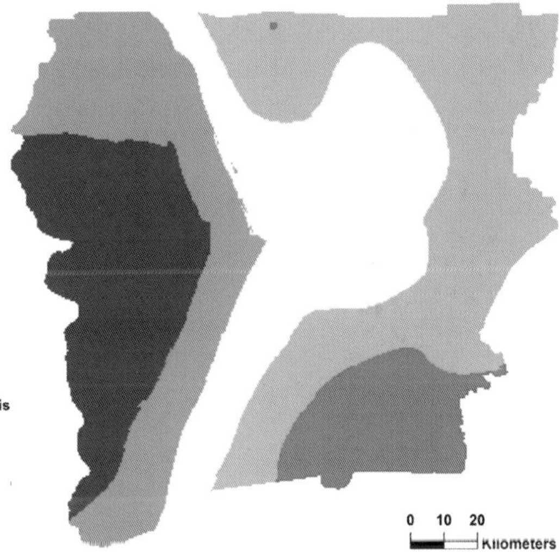

Figure 3.0 Association between rainfall and bacterial meningitis incidence in the Upper West Region 2018–2020
Source: Field Data

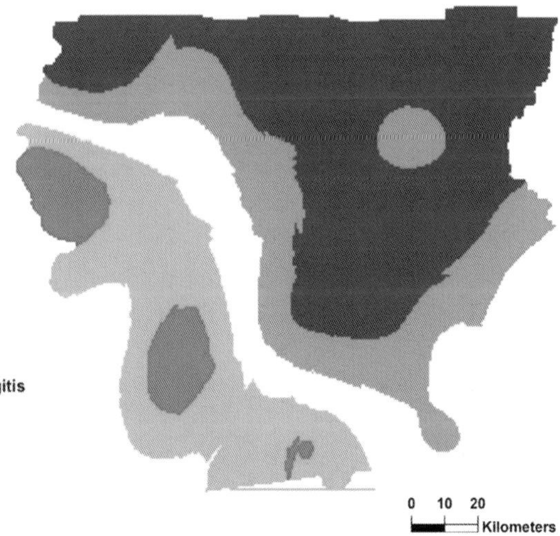

Figure 4.0 Association between wind speed and bacterial meningitis incidence in the Upper West Region 2018–2020
Source: Field Data

#04.1 Ghana
Spatial Epidemiology of Bacterial Meningitis in the Upper West Region of Ghana: The Effect of Climate Change on the Disease Burden

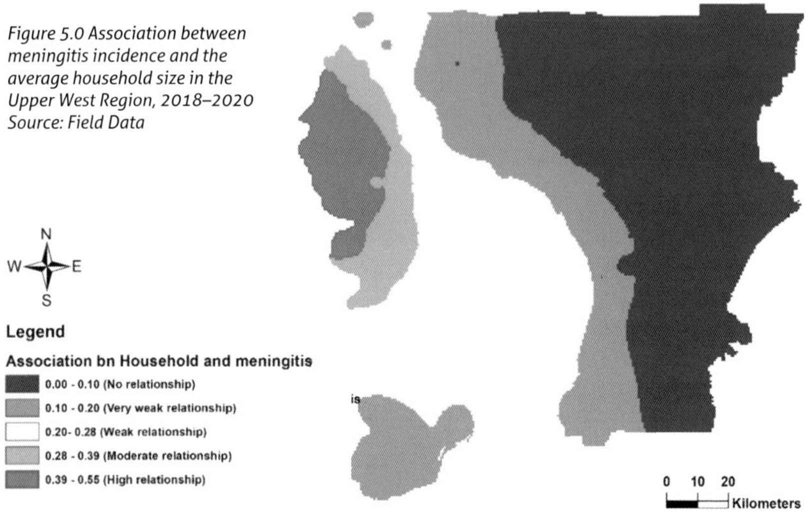

Figure 5.0 Association between meningitis incidence and the average household size in the Upper West Region, 2018–2020
Source: Field Data

Other researchers have also described how socioeconomic dynamics determine the interplay between population and disease dynamics (Dukić et al., 2012a; Mazamay et al., 2020a). The current study sought to understand how household size influences the prevalence of meningitis. Since this disease is contagious and can also be transmitted through personal contact and droplets from the nose and throat (Nii et al., 2014), the study hypothesized that the household size had no significant impact on the prevalence of meningitis. Interestingly, the results indicate that there exists a positive association between the size of a household and the prevalence of meningitis (R2 = 0.56; AICCs = 598). The OLS predicted weakly about the association (R2 = 0.14; AICCs = 599) indicating that weighted regression provided a robust predictive power. However, after careful inspection of Figure 5.0, the local geographically weighted regression model reveals that the relationship is not uniform across the region; a very high relationship class was observed at the Northwestern flank while the low to very low relationship class was observed at the central and eastern sides.

SOCIO-CLIMATIC EFFECT ON MENINGITIS IN UPPER WEST REGION OF GHANA.

Meningitis remains one of the draconian global public health burdens. Considering already deplorable economic, social, and environmental conditions in Sub-Sahara Africa, the incidence of meningitis has considerably disrupted healthcare systems and claimed many lives. For example in the Democratic Republic of Congo, 118,378 incidences of meningitis were recorded by the Ministry of Health between 2000 and 2018 of which the lethality exceeded 10% (Mazamay et al., 2020b). However, distribution was highly variable, as Kinshasa recorded the highest. Regarding the heterogeneous nature of the disease distribution spatially, coupled with changing nature of the bio-climatic conditions, researchers have described various social and environmental conditions influencing this epidemic in the meningitis belt, spanning Ethiopia to Senegal (Meentemeyer et al., 2011). However, some nations in the meningitis belt have been neglected even though prevalence has been noted to be higher as well; for example between 18 and 200 per 100,000 people contracted meningitis per annum (between 2010–2011) in most populated areas in Nigeria (Abdussalam et al., 2014a). It is however unclear how the changing environmental and social factors affect meningitis, especially in Ghana which is equally noted to record higher annual cases of the epidemic (Kwarteng et al., 2017a; Nii et al., 2014). In this study, we relied on geographically weighted regression to understand how wind speed, rainfall, and household sizes affect meningitis cases differentially across space in the Upper West Region. It was found that, based on the Global weighted regression model, the prevalence of meningitis was better explained inversely by rainfall ($R2 = 0.93$; AICCs = 510.87) as opposed to the Ordinary Least Squares ($R2 = 0.27$; AICCs = 584.16). The study demonstrated that, through the local geographic regression model, the association between meningitis prevalence and precipitation does not follow a homogenous spatial order, but varies significantly (see Figure 3.0), and will therefore aid in the development of targetable policy.

Similarly, a significant negative association between rainfall and meningitis has been reported in other studies. For example, in a study conducted by (Abdussalam et al., 2014; Dukić et al., 2012) in the North-western part of Nigeria, it was discovered that rainfall though may increase in the future, will have no perceptible impact on meningitis epidemics. This corroborated other studies such as a study conducted by (Ayanlade et al., 2020) where moisture condition is associated inversely with meningitis incidence. Even though comparing Figures 2.0 and 3.0, areas of high prevalence had almost negative to no relationship with rainfall, effective bio-climatic maintenance will still be needed to increase rainfall amount in the future to reduce meningitis prevalence. This may include integrating afforestation projects into health intervention policy to increase rainfall amounts in the region. It was also found that, based on the global geographic weighted regression model (GGWR), wind speed on the contrary had a stronger positive influence on meningitis cases (R2 = 0.80; AICCs = 668) than the ordinary least squares (R2 = 0.07; AICCs = 601.72). Comparing Figures 2.0 and 4.0, it is apparent that the association between meningitis and wind speed was stronger where the prevalence was also high and got spatially weaker towards the middle part of the region where people have sparingly settled. This is reasonable because arguably, droplets of these bacteria can be transmitted under higher surface wind speed conditions (Sultan et al., 2005b). A study conducted in Ghana by (Sultan et al., 2005) confirmed that surface wind speed showed a clear linkage between population dynamics of diseases and climate. This may explain why places in the higher latitudinal regions experience fewer meningitis cases compared to areas closer to the equator (Abdussalam et al., 2014b; Dukić et al., 2012a). Given the ecological nature of the Upper West Region where wind speed is high and dust is pervasive, it raises considerable concern about the future dynamics of meningitis incidence. Natural-based Interventions such as afforestation that may help to increase wind density and reduce wind speed and specks of dust will be helpful to attenuate this epidemic prevalence. Other researchers have also described how socioeconomic dynamics determine the interplay between population and disease dynamics (Dukić et al., 2012a; Mazamay et al., 2020a). This current study sought to understand how household size for instance influences the prevalence. Since this disease is communicable and can also be transmitted through personal contact and droplets from the nose and throat (Nii et al., 2014), The study hypothesized that the size household had no significant impact on the prevalence of meningitis. Results indicate that there exists a positive association between the size of a household and the prevalence of meningitis (R2 = 0.56; AICCs = 598) even though the OLS predicted weakly about the association (R2 = 0.14; AICCs = 599) indicating that weighted regression provided a robust predictive power. However, after careful inspection of Figure 5.0, the local geographically weighted regression model reveals that the relationship is not uniform across the region; a very high relationship class was observed at the Northwestern flank while the low to very low relationship class was observed at the central and eastern sides. This heterogeneity is reasonable since the eastern side is sparsely settled. This may explain why meningitis outbreaks have been higher in urban areas in Congo and Nigeria (Abdussalam et al., 2014b; Amegah et al., 2016; Mazamay et al., 2020a). Besides the high probability of spread of spatial mobility and higher population density (Nii et al., 2014). A poor economic situation such as poverty, malnutrition, and overcrowding among the urban poor may exacerbate the incidence of the diseases (Mazamay et al., 2020a) which is very obvious from this current study. This study relied on one dimension of the socio-economic situation; therefore, a more precise and holistic socio-economic well-being and equality index model development may better reveal an augmented reality about the situation of meningitis in the Upper West Region. Future research will therefore benefit greatly from considering a comprehensive characterization of the socio-economic condition of people and how it impacts meningitis transmission and spatial diffusion in Ghana. This, however, may not be achievable if a well-defined policy is not formulated, as currently, no such policy is available solely for meningitis (Dukić et al., 2012a). Amid Covid-19, attention has even shifted from this epidemic; consequently, continued neglect coupled with the poor socio-economic condition may worsen the situation of meningitis in the Upper West(Ali et al., 2022b). It has also been discovered latitude also plays a significant factor in meningitis prevalence in many regions across the world (Mazamay et al., 2020a), the study did not consider that due to the smaller spatial extent of the study. However, for national policy against the epidemic, it will be highly beneficial to incorporate this factor to leverage spatial targeting and intervention effort.

CONCLUSION. Based on the evidence, bacterial meningitis exhibits a non-random distribution. Identifying the geographical and socio-bioclimatic risk factors responsible for spatial patterns of meningitis prevalence is a vital step in eradicating the disease. Yearly rainfall was found to have an inverse relationship with disease prevalence. Higher levels of rainfall lower the incidence of the disease by minimizing atmospheric dust and temperature, both of which aid in the spread of meningitis. Household size was significantly associated with the spread of meningitis, with the relationship being non-uniform across the region. A high relationship class was observed at the north-western flank.—

REFERENCES

Abdussalam, A. F., Monaghan, A. J., Steinhoff, D. F., Dukic, V. M., Hayden, M. H., Hopson, T. M., Thornes, J. E., & Leckebusch, G. C. (2014a). The impact of climate change on meningitis in northwest Nigeria: An assessment using CMIP5 climate model simulations. Weather, Climate, and Society, 6(3), 371–379. https://doi.org/10.1175/WCAS-D-13-00068.1 • Abdussalam, A. F., Monaghan, A. J., Steinhoff, D. F., Dukic, V. M., Hayden, M. H., Hopson, T. M., Thornes, J. E., & Leckebusch, G. C. (2014b). The impact of climate change on meningitis in northwest Nigeria: An assessment using CMIP5 climate model simulations. Weather, Climate, and Society, 6(3), 371–379. https://doi.org/10.1175/

#04.1 Ghana
Spatial Epidemiology of Bacterial Meningitis in the Upper West Region of Ghana: The Effect of Climate Change on the Disease Burden

WCAS-D-13-00068.1 • AJ Pollard. (2004). Global epidemiology of meningococcal disease and vaccine efficacy. The Pediatric Infectious. • Aku, F., Lessa, F., ... F. A.-B.-MMWR. M. and, & 2017, U. (2017). Meningitis outbreak caused by vaccine-preventable bacterial pathogens—northern Ghana, 2016. Ncbi.Nlm.Nih.Gov. • Ali, M., Moses, A., Nakua, E. K., Punguyire, D., Cheabu, B. S. N., Avevor, P. M., & Basit, K. A. (2022a). Spatial epidemiology of bacterial meningitis in the Upper West Region of Ghana: Analysis of disease surveillance data 2018–2020. Clinical Infection in Practice, 16, 100160. https://doi.org/10.1016/J.CLINPR.2022.100160 • Ali, M., Moses, A., Nakua, E. K., Punguyire, D., Cheabu, B. S. N., Avevor, P. M., & Basit, K. A. (2022b). Spatial epidemiology of bacterial meningitis in the Upper West Region of Ghana: Analysis of disease surveillance data 2018–2020. Clinical Infection in Practice, 16, 100160. https://doi.org/10.1016/J.CLINPR.2022.100160 • AM, M., & MC Thomson. (2002). Where is the meningitis belt? Defining an area at risk of epidemic meningitis in Africa. Academic.Oup.Com. • Amegah, A. K., Rezza, G., & Jaakkola, J. J. K. (2016). Temperature-related morbidity and mortality in Sub-Saharan Africa: A systematic review of the empirical evidence. In Environment International (Vol. 91, pp. 133–149). Elsevier Ltd. https://doi.org/10.1016/j.envint.2016.02.027 • Asori, M., Musah, A., & Gyasi, R. (2022). Bio-climatic Impact on malaria prevalence in Ghana: A multi-scale spatial Modeling. African Geographical Review. https://doi.org/10.1080/19376812.2022.2130378 • Asori, M., Musah, A., & Peprah, P. (2022). Spatial targeting and prediction of factors responsible for optimum Covid-19 based social distancing – the case of Upper west region, Ghana. In ResearchSquare. https://doi.org/10.21203/rs.3.rs-1364371 • Ayanlade, A., Sergi, C., & Ayanlade, O. S. (2020). Malaria and meningitis under climate change: initial assessment of climate information service in Nigeria. Meteorological Applications, 27(5), 1–11. https://doi.org/10.1002/met.1953 • Carod Artal, F. J. (2015). Meningococcal meningitis: vaccination outbreak response and epidemiological changes in the African meningitis belt. International Health, 7(4), 226–227. https://doi.org/10.1093/inthealth/ihv025 • CDC. (2016). Laboratory Methods for the Diagnosis of Meningitis - CHAPTER 2: Epi. 1–8. • Domo, N. R., Nuolabong, C., Nyarko, K. M., Kenu, E., Balagumyetime, P., Konnyebal, G., Noora, C. L., Ameme, K. D., Wurapa, F., & Afari, E. (2017). Uncommon mixed outbreak of pneumococcal and meningococcal meningitis in Jirapa District, Upper West Region, Ghana, 2016. Ghana Medical Journal, 51(4), 149–155. https://doi.org/10.4314/gmj.v51i4.2 • Dukić, V., Hayden, M., Forgor, A. A., Hopson, T., Akweongo, P., Hodgson, A., Monaghan, A., Wiedinmyer, C., Yoksas, T., Thomson, M. C., Trzaska, S., & Pandya, R. (2012a). The Role of Weather in Meningitis Outbreaks in Navrongo, Ghana: A Generalized Additive Modeling Approach. Journal of Agricultural, Biological, and Environmental Statistics, 17(3), 442–460. https://doi.org/10.1007/s13253-012-0095-9 • Dukić, V., Hayden, M., Forgor, A. A., Hopson, T., Akweongo, P., Hodgson, A., Monaghan, A., Wiedinmyer, C., Yoksas, T., Thomson, M. C., Trzaska, S., & Pandya, R. (2012b). The Role of Weather in Meningitis Outbreaks in Navrongo, Ghana: A Generalized Additive Modeling Approach. Journal of Agricultural, Biological, and Environmental Statistics, 17(3), 442–460. https://doi.org/10.1007/s13253-012-0095-9 • Edward, H. (2020). The history of meningitis. Meningitis Research Foundation. • Ferraro, C. F., Trotter, C. L., Nascimento, M. C., Jusot, J. F., Omotara, B. A., Hodgson, A., Ali, O., Alavo, S., Sow, S., Daugla, D. M., & Stuart, J. M. (2014). Household crowding, social mixing patterns and respiratory symptoms in seven countries of the African meningitis belt. PLoS ONE, 9(7). https://doi.org/10.1371/JOURNAL.PONE.0101129 • GHS. (2020). Annual Health Performance Report, Upper West Region. • GSS. (2020). Ghana Population and Housing Census. • Hodgson, A., Smith, T., ... S. G.-T. of the, & 2001, undefined. (2001). Risk factors for meningococcal meningitis in northern Ghana. Academic.Oup.Com, 95, 477–480. • IDSR-GHS. (2019). Technical Guidelines for IDSR in Ghana. In Booklet Six: Vol. Section 11. • Joseph, S. J., Topaz, N., Chang, H.-Y., Whaley, M. J., Vuong, J. T., Chen, A., Hu, F., Schmink, S. E., Jenkins, L. T., Rodriguez-Rivera, L. D., Thomas, J. D., Acosta, A. M., McNamara, L., Soeters, H. M., Mbaeyi, S., & Wang, X. (2020). Insights on Population Structure and Within-Host Genetic Changes among Meningococcal Carriage Isolates from U.S. Universities. MSphere, 5(2). https://doi.org/10.1128/msphere.00197-20 • Kwarteng, A., Amuasi, J., Annan, A., Ahuno, S., Opare, D., Nagel, M., Vinnemeier, C., May, J., & Owusu-Dabo, E. (2017a). Current meningitis outbreak in Ghana: Historical perspectives and the importance of diagnostics. Acta Tropica, 169, 51–56. https://doi.org/10.1016/j.actatropica.2017.01.014 • Kwarteng, A., Amuasi, J., Annan, A., Ahuno, S., Opare, D., Nagel, M., Vinnemeier, C., May, J., & Owusu-Dabo, E. (2017b). Current meningitis outbreak in Ghana: Historical perspectives and the importance of diagnostics. Acta Tropica, 169, 51–56. https://doi.org/10.1016/j.actatropica.2017.01.014 • Mansour, S., Al, A., Al-said, A., & Al-said, A. (2020). Since January 2020 Elsevier has created a COVID-19 resource centre with free information in English and Mandarin on the novel coronavirus COVID- 19 . The COVID-19 resource centre is hosted on Elsevier Connect , the company ' s public news and information . January. • Mazamay, S., Broutin, H., Bompangue, D., Muyembe, J. J., & Guégan, J. F. (2020a). The environmental drivers of bacterial meningitis epidemics in the democratic republic of congo, central africa. PLoS Neglected Tropical Diseases, 14(10), 1–16. https://doi.org/10.1371/journal.pntd.0008634 • Mazamay, S., Broutin,

H., Bompangue, D., Muyembe, J. J., & Guégan, J. F. (2020b). The environmental drivers of bacterial meningitis epidemics in the democratic republic of congo, central africa. PLoS Neglected Tropical Diseases, 14(10), 1–16. https://doi.org/10.1371/journal.pntd.0008634 • Meentemeyer, R. K., Haas, S. E., & Václavík, T. (2011). Landscape Epidemiology of Emerging Infectious Diseases in Natural and Human-Altered Ecosystems. Http://Dx.Doi.Org/10.1146/Annurev-Phyto-081211-172938, 50, 379–402. https://doi.org/10.1146/ANNUREV-PHYTO-081211-172938 • Nii, S., Codjoe, A., & Nabie, V. A. (2014). Climate Change and Cerebrospinal Meningitis in the Ghanaian Meningitis Belt. International Journal of Environmental Research and Public Health, 11, 6923–6939. https://doi.org/10.3390/ijerph110706923 • Paireau, J., Girond, F., Collard, J. M., Maïnassara, H. B., & Jusot, J. F. (2012). Analysing spatio-temporal clustering of meningococcal meningitis outbreaks in Niger Reveals opportunities for improved disease control. PLoS Neglected Tropical Diseases, 6(3). https://doi.org/10.1371/journal.pntd.0001577 • Putz, K., Hayani, K., Practice, F. Z.-C. C. in O., & 2013, U. (2013). Meningitis. Primarycare.Theclinics.Com. • Souza, S., Costa, M., ... J. P.-R. da S., & 2012, U. (2012). Bacterial meningitis and living conditions. SciELO Brasil. • Sultan, B., Labadi, K., Guégan, J. F., & Janicot, S. (2005a). Climate drives the meningitis epidemics onset in West Africa. PLoS Medicine, 2(1), 0043–0049. https://doi.org/10.1371/journal.pmed.0020006 • Sultan, B., Labadi, K., Guégan, J. F., & Janicot, S. (2005b). Climate drives the meningitis epidemics onset in West Africa. PLoS Medicine, 2(1), 0043–0049. https://doi.org/10.1371/journal.pmed.0020006 • Tikhomirova, E., Santamariab, M., & Estevesc, K. (1997). Meningococcal disease: public health burden and control. In apps.who.int. • van Donkelaar, A., Martin, R. v, Brauer, M., Hsu, N. C., Kahn, R. A., Levy, R. C., Lyapustin, A., Sayer, A. M., & winker, D. M. (2018). Global Annual PM2.5 Grids from MODIS, MISR and SeaWiFS Aerosol Optical Depth (AOD) with GWR, 1998-2016. NASA Socioeconomic Data and Applications Center (SEDAC). https://doi.org/10.7927/H4ZK5DQS • WHO. (1997). Control of epidemic meningococcal disease. WHO practical guidelines. 2nd edition. Journal of the Irish Dental Association, 19(5), 203–205. • WHO. (2011a). Meningitis Weekly Bulletin. Meningvax.Org, 1–10. • WHO. (2011b). Meningococcal vaccines: WHO position paper, November 2011. Releve Epidemiologique Hebdomadaire, 86(47), 521–539. • WHO. (2018). Meningococcal Meningitis. • WHO. (2020). Meningococcal Meningitis Facts. WHO. https://www.who.int/news-room/fact-sheets/detail/meningococcal-meningitis • WHO. (2021). Meningitis Fact Sheet. https://www.who.int/news-room/fact-sheets/detail/meningitis

AUTHORS

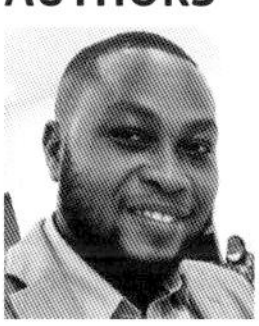

Musah Ali - BSc, MPhil
Kwame Nkrumah University of Science and Technology / Ghana Health Service
Department of Epidemiology and Biostatistics
Tel: +233244730080 | E-mail: bamwara.ma@gmail.com

Asori Moses – BA, PhD (Student)
University of North Carolina, Charlotte, USA
Department of Geography and Earth Science,
Tel: +19803370479 | E-mail: masori@uncc.edu

Prof. Emmanuel K. Nakua - BSc, MSc, PGDiploma, PhD
Kwame Nkrumah University of Science and Technology
Department of Epidemiology and Biostatistics
Tel: +233246517578 | E-mail: emmanngh@gmail.com / enakua.chs@knust.edu.gh

#04.2 Ghana
Prediction models for the composite outcome of heart failure and stroke among persons with hypertension and type 2 diabetes in Ghana

Robert Asampong, Yeetey Enuameh, Emmanuel Kweku Nakua, Gabriel Asare Okyere, John Humphrey Amuasi, Fred Stephen Sarfo

ABSTRACT. BACKGROUND. Persons with Hypertension and type 2 diabetes (T2D) are at risk of developing major adverse cardiovascular events such as heart failure and stroke. In Ghana, evidence on the incidence rate and clinically relevant predictors of these two adverse cardiovascular events in such persons is low. We sought to determine the incidence rate and develop prediction models for the composite outcome of heart failure and stroke among this at-risk population.

METHODS. This was a prospective cohort study involving persons with hypertension and T2D aged 18 years and above across five public hospitals. Participants were followed up every two months for 18 months during which they were clinically assessed for first-ever heart failure or stroke. We examined the predictive effect of 27 factors on the composite outcome using the Least Absolute Shrinkage and Selection Operator (LASSO) and the backward-stepwise regression methods for Cox proportional hazards. The models were evaluated using Harrell's concordance index (c-index).

RESULTS. A total of 3214 participants [mean age (standard deviation): 57.4 (±12.7) years; females (76.9%)] were included in the analysis. At the end of follow-up, 15 incident heart failures and 54 incident strokes occurred, resulting in an overall incidence rate of 14.49 (95% CI: 11.44–18.34) per 1000 person-years. From the LASSO model, male gender, being unemployed, past smoker, duration of hypertension/T2D, triglycerides at enrolment, previous diagnosis with high cholesterol, previous diagnosis with a heart attack, haemoglobin A1c (HbA1c), and body mass index (BMI) were predictive of the composite outcome (c-index: 0.79). The backward-stepwise model selected age (HR=1.03, 95% CI: 1.01–1.05), male gender (HR=2.11, 95% CI: 1.26–3.54), BMI (HR=1.37, 95% CI: 1.01–1.85), previous diagnosis with a heart attack (HR=2.36, 95% CI: 1.29–4.32), and triglycerides at enrolment (HR=1.75, 95% CI: 1.49–2.06) as the predictors (c-index: 0.74).

CONCLUSION. Among Ghanaians with hypertension and T2D, the incidence of heart failure and stroke is moderately high. The identified predictors could inform a more focused health education and counselling plan, and enhanced monitoring of lipid profiles of at-risk persons.

KEYWORDS. heart failure, stroke, hypertension, type 2 diabetes, prediction model

INTRODUCTION. Heart failure and stroke are among the major cardiovascular events (MACE) of medical and public health concern worldwide. Evidence shows that hypertension and diabetes mellitus are among the leading underlying risk factors of these adverse cardiovascular outcomes [1–3]. In the global south, the burden of hypertension and diabetes is on the ascendency, and this has dire implications on the incidence of heart failure and stroke [4]. Moreover, these adverse outcomes negatively impact quality of life and significantly contribute to disability, hospitalisations, and mortality [5–7]. However, the estimation of the incidence rate and identification of clinically relevant predictors of these two adverse cardiovascular outcomes are challenged by the inadequacy of robust prospective studies in resource-poor settings.

Worldwide, the incidence of heart failure has stabilized and is reportedly declining in high-income countries [8–11]. However, its prevalence is rising as a result of a demographic transition and an increase in ageing populations [9, 12]. As reported in a global study, heart failure occurs in over 64 million people globally (8.52 per 1000 population) [10, 11]. In 2020, heart failure accounted for 9.9 million years lost due to disability [10].

The global population-based incidence of strokes on the other hand has moderately declined over the past two decades according to the Global and Regional Burden of Disease (GBD) report [13]. Despite this downward trend, the annual absolute cases, the mortality counts and the disability-adjusted life years (DALYs) have increased significantly [3, 13]. Within the African context, however, relatively few studies have assessed the incidence rate of heart failure and stroke. Akinyemi et al. [14] in 2019 reported that the magnitude of haemorrhagic stroke ranges from 15% in Kenya to as high as 41% in Ethiopia. A review by Owolabi and colleagues [15] in 2018 also found that stroke incidence ranged from 25 per 100,000 person-years (py) in Nigeria to 250 per 100,000 py in Egypt. Most of these studies however did not assess sub-groups such as persons with hypertension and diabetes who are at a greater risk of developing these adverse outcomes. As a result, the estimates from these studies are not truly representative of, nor generalizable to persons with hypertension and/or diabetes. In Ghana, only a few published studies have assessed incident heart failure or stroke as an adverse outcome among persons with hypertension and diabetes in Ghana [16–18]. Efforts to mitigate these adverse outcomes have also not seen much progress [19]. Without substantial empirical evidence, the dynamics of these adverse outcomes and their possible predictors remain to be adequately understood, and will further make current interventions only achieve suboptimal results. Although Sarfo and colleagues [16] in 2018 found that the incidence of stroke among Ghanaians with hypertension and diabetes was 14.2 per 1000 py, no further studies have examined stroke and heart failure as composite outcomes. The aim of this study, therefore, was to estimate the incidence rate, and develop predictive models for the composite outcome of heart failure and stroke among persons with hypertension and T2D in Ghana. This study contributes important scientific evidence that is relevant to clinical practice and public health action.

METHODS

Study design and settings

The present study was based on data from the Ghana Affordability and Access Program (GAAP). A prospective cohort design was employed to collect data on baseline characteristics, biochemical profile, cardiovascular, cerebrovascular, and renal outcomes every two (2) months for eighteen (18) months. The study was conducted in five public health facilities that provide hypertension and diabetes services including diagnosis and management in Ghana. The facilities were located in the central forest, northern savanna, mixed zone, and coastal savanna ecological zones of Ghana. The administrative regions and their corresponding study facilities are as follows: Northern Region (Tamale Teaching Hospital (TTH) and Kings Medical Centre (KMC); Ashanti Region (Komfo Anokye Teaching Hospital and Agogo Presbyterian District Hospital); and Eastern Region (Atua Government Hospital).

Study population, recruitment and follow-up

This study involved persons aged 18 years or older with old or newly diagnosed hypertension and/or type 2 diabetes, and presenting for routine care and management at the facilities. After obtaining written informed consent, study participants were recruited and followed up. Those that were unstable or symptomatic with a hypertensive or diabetic emergency requiring hospitalization were excluded. During clinic registration or attendance of persons with a diagnosis of diabetes or hypertension, trained research assistants approached them to participate in the study. Participants were then recruited into the study by following a standardized methodology established for the study. Privacy and confidentiality were ensured during the entire recruitment process. Patient enrolment began in July 2014. By May 2015, a total of 3300 participants were recruited. The study was completed on June 30, 2017.

Data collection

Data on demographic, lifestyle and behavioural characteristics were collected through face-to-face interviews using a structured questionnaire. Anthropometric measures of height, weight, and waist circumference were taken by nurses at the study sites at enrolment. Detailed medical history was also extracted from the medical records of all study participants. Samples of venous blood were taken by trained phlebotomists at all study sites for biochemical analysis. Specific data on cardiovascular outcomes, blood pressure control, blood sugar control, and biochemical profile were collected at two intervals for a total follow-up time of 18 months. For persons that were lost to follow-up, research assistants followed up to inquire about the cause.

Data quality assurance and quality control

To ensure that data were of high quality, research assistants were specially trained before the commencement of the study. Standardization and uniformity across all study sites were ensured by contracting an International Organization for Standardization (ISO)-certified and quality-assured laboratory to undertake all biochemical panels and analyses.

Variables

The main outcomes (primary endpoints) in this study were incident heart failure or stroke as defined according to the International Classification of Diseases (ICD-10). For this composite outcome, the survival time of whichever event occurred first was used for the analysis. Participants who did not have any of the outcomes were right-censored. The predictor variables for this study included sociodemographic characteristics, medical history, biochemical profile, anthropometric measurements, and lifestyle factors.

Statistical analysis

The data were cleaned and exported to R Studio for statistical analysis. Missing baseline data were handled with multiple imputations using chained random forests. Descriptive statistics were performed for all variables. Kaplan-Meier non-parametric survival curves were used to illustrate the survival probability. Log-rank tests were used to test the categorical differences in survival function at 5% significance level. Prediction analysis for the identification of background and clinical predictors was conducted using the Least Absolute Shrinkage and Selection Operator (LASSO) method for Cox proportional hazards regression. A 10-fold cross-validation framework was employed in building the model and the tuning parameters used were $\alpha=1$ and an appropriate choice of lambda (λ) from the cross-validation plot. A backward-stepwise elimination method was also used to identify the predictors. Results from the stepwise model are presented in a forest plot. Predictive accuracies of the models were evaluated using Harrell's concordance index (c-index)[20].

#04.2 Ghana
Prediction models for the composite outcome of heart failure and stroke among hypertension and type 2 diabetes patients in Ghana

Ethical considerations

Ethical review and approval for this research project were obtained from the Committee on Human Research, Publications, and Ethics (CHRPE) of the Kwame Nkrumah University of Science and Technology (CHRPE/AP/298/14) and the Ghana Health Service Ethical Review Committee (GHS-ERC: 12/07/14).

RESULTS

Sociodemographic characteristics of study participants

Table 1 presents the baseline socio-demographic characteristics of study participants. There were 3214 participants overall (mean age (±standard deviation) was 57(±12.7) years). More than half, 1809 (56.3%), of participants were below 60 years, and the majority 2473 (76.9%) were females. More than a third of participants, 1201 (37.4%), had no formal education whereas only 569 (17.7%) had had secondary school education. In the preceding 12 months, most participants 1372 (42.7%), were self-employed or engaged in their own business whereas 338 (10.5%) were involved in government or private company work, 846 (26.3%), were unemployed and 242 (7.5%) were retirees. There were also more urban dwellers 1402

Variable	No stroke/Heart failure (n=3145)	Stroke/heart failure (n=69)	Total study sample (n=3214)
Mean age (SD) *years*			57.4 (±12.7)
Age category			
Below 60 years	1778 (57)	31 (45)	1809 (56.3)
60 years and above	1367 (43)	38 (55)	1405 (43.7)
Gender			
Female	2428 (77)	45 (65)	2473 (76.9)
Male	717 (23)	24 (35)	741 (23.1)
Highest level of education			
No formal education	1177 (37)	24 (35)	1201 (37.4)
Basic school	1060 (34)	23 (33)	1083 (33.7)
Secondary school	554 (18)	15 (22)	569 (17.7)
Tertiary	354 (11)	7 (10)	361 (11.2)
Work status (past 12 months)			
Government/Private	331 (11)	7 (10)	338 (10.5)
Self-employed	1353 (43)	19 (28)	1372 (42.7)
Farmer	407 (13)	9 (13)	416 (13.0)
Retired	238 (7)	4 (6)	242 (7.5)
Unemployed	816 (26)	30 (43)	846 (26.3)
Settlement			
Rural	1066 (33)	19 (28)	1085 (33.8)
Peri-urban	708 (23)	19 (28)	727 (22.6)
Urban	1371 (44)	31 (44)	1402 (43.6)

Table 1: Socio-demographic characteristics of study participants

(43.6%) than those residents in rural and peri-urban areas.

Incidence rate and survival of the composite outcome of heart failure or stroke

For the composite outcome of heart failure or stroke, the overall incidence rate was 14.49 per 1000 py. Higher incidence rates were observed among males and participants aged 60 years and above.
The overall survival probability for the composite outcome of heart failure or stroke was 0.979.

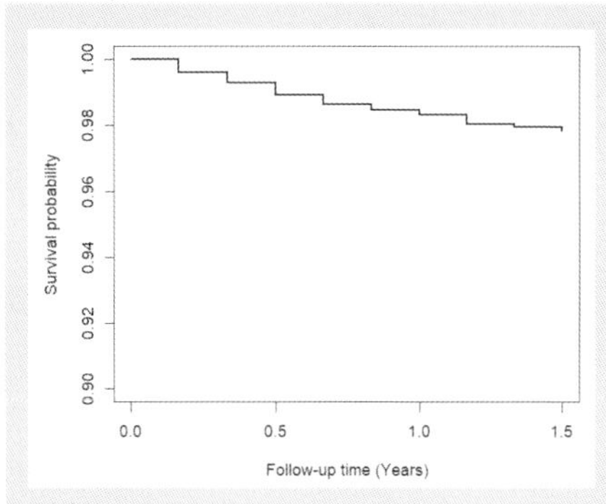

Figure 1: Kaplan-Meier survival curve for the composite outcome

Background and clinical predictors of the composite outcome of heart failure or stroke

Table 3 presents the background and clinical predictors selected via the LASSO model. Ten (10) predictors were selected of which three (3) were background characteristics. Male gender (β=0.3542) and being unemployed (β=0.1394) were associated with a greater predicted risk of the composite outcome. Also, being a past smoker emerged as a strong predictor of having either of the two outcomes (β=0.2764). Except for T2D which was associated with a lower predicted risk (β = -0.1338), the remainder of the selected clinical predictors were associated with a higher predicted risk (β>0) of the composite outcome. These predictors include BMI (β=0.0452) and having ever been diagnosed with high cholesterol (β=0.0428) or heart attack (β=0.2456). For each one-year increase in the disease status of participants and one unit increase in HbA1c at enrolment, slightly high predicted risks of the composite outcome were observed (β¬=0.0162) and (β=0.0214) respectively. For the LASSO model, the corresponding c-index was 0.79 indicating good model performance in predicting individual risk of the composite outcome.
Similar predictors, although fewer, were identified using the backward-stepwise method (Figure 2). The predictors which were the most predictive of the composite outcome were age (HR= 1.03, 95% CI: 1.01–1.05), gender (male) (HR=2.11, 95% CI: 1.26–3.54), BMI (HR=1.37, 95% CI: 1.01–1.85), previous diagnosis with a heart attack (HR=2.36, 95% CI: 1.29–4.32), and triglyceride (mmol/L) at enrolment (HR=1.75, 95% CI: 1.49–2.06). The c-index of this model was 0.74.

#04.2 Ghana
Prediction models for the composite outcome of heart failure and stroke among hypertension and type 2 diabetes patients in Ghana

Variable	Heart failure/Stroke IR (95% CI) per 1000 PY	Log-rank test: χ^2 (p-value)
Overall	14.49 (11.44–18.34)	
Age category		
Below 60 years	11.55 (8.12–16.42)	
60 years and above	18.34 (13.35–25.21)	**3.72 (0.054)**
Gender		
Male	22.05 (14.78–32.89)	
Female	12.27 (9.16–16.44)	**5.50 (0.019)** *
Disease status		
Hypertension	14.17 (10.31–19.47)	
T2D	7.99 (3.33–19.20)	
Hypertension and T2D	17.90 (12.19–26.29)	**3.00 (0.223)**

*IR: Incidence rate; CI: Confidence interval; PY: Person-years; * Significant categorical difference in survivor function at α=0.05*

Table 2: Incidence rate of the composite outcome by age category, gender, and disease status

	LASSO coefficients
Background predictors	
Gender (Male)	0.3542
Work status (Unemployed)	0.1394
Past smoker	0.2764
Clinical predictors	
Disease status (T2D only)	-0.1338
Duration of HPT/T2D/BOTH	0.0162
Triglycerides	0.5860
Ever diagnosed with high cholesterol	0.0428
Ever diagnosed with a heart attack	0.2456
HbA1c at enrolment	0.0214
BMI	0.0452
C-index: 0.79	

Table 3: Background and clinical predictors of the composite outcome

DISCUSSION. We estimated the incidence rate of the composite outcome of heart failure or stroke and examined their possible predictors. To the best of our knowledge, this is the first study in Ghana to provide evidence of the composite occurrence of these adverse outcomes among persons with hyper-

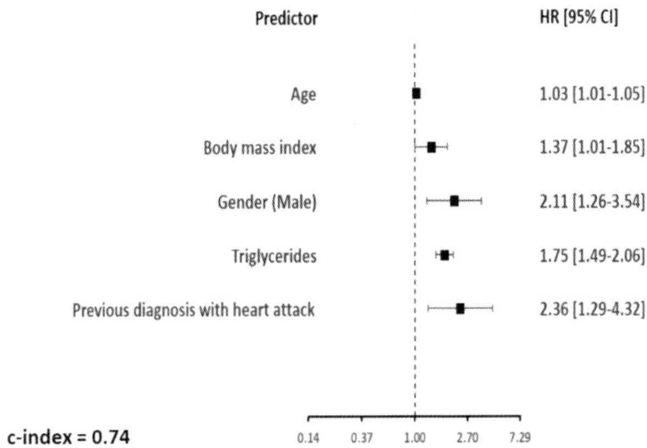

Figure 2: Predictors of the composite outcome of heart failure or stroke

tension and diabetes. In this analysis, the overall incidence rate was 14.49 (95% CI: 11.44–18.34) per 1000 py. The estimate is however lower than the 20.41 per 1000 py reported among persons with HIV in Ghana [17]. This disparity could be due to the evidence of direct infection of cardiac myocytes in persons with HIV. Additionally, reduction of CD4 T-cells among persons with HIV has been associated with increased risk of atherosclerotic cardiac events, and this may have contributed to the relatively high incidence rate in that study [17, 21]. We find that heart failure and stroke are fast becoming crucial contributors to morbidity among persons with hypertension and diabetes, with stroke in particular at the forefront. In this study, males had higher predicted risk of the composite outcome of heart failure or stroke. Evidence across the literature however shows conflicting findings. Ntiyani et al. [22] for instance reported that stroke risk is higher among females than males. However, it can be argued that among males, higher uptake of unhealthy lifestyles and behaviours such as smoking, excessive alcohol intake, medication non-adherence, and poor health-seeking practices could predispose them to incident heart failure or stroke. A counterargument for the previously observed higher risk among females is that they are more likely to present with multimorbidities such as hypercholesterolaemia, diabetes, overweight, obesity, and hypertension according to Jenča et al. (2021), and these may predispose them to the development of heart failure or stroke.

#04.2 Ghana
Prediction models for the composite outcome of heart failure and stroke among hypertension and type 2 diabetes patients in Ghana

Being unemployed was also found to be highly predictive of incident heart failure or stroke in the LASSO model. This finding is in congruity with updated evidence by the American Heart Association [24] and the results of a systematic review in Morocco [25]. The finding also has implications for the Universal Health Coverage target to ensure financial risk protection for the poor and vulnerable, which includes the unemployed. Similarly, being a past smoker was found to be predictive of the composite outcome. This is consistent with previous studies in Botswana and Ethiopia [22, 26].

Regarding the clinical predictors, the duration of hypertension and/or diabetes was found to be associated with a slightly high predicted risk of the composite outcome. The finding corroborates prior evidence from elsewhere [22, 27, 28]. The study by Mefford et al. (2020) among both black and white adults also found a similar association. Furthermore, prolonged uncontrolled hypertension is likely to lead to right ventricular hypertrophy and this has been associated with incident heart failure [30]. The same condition also increases the risk of stroke; especially haemorrhagic stroke [13, 15].

In addition, previous diagnosis with high cholesterol and having high triglycerides at baseline were found to be associated with a greater risk of developing the composite outcome. The relationship between these risk factors and heart failure or stroke has been observed in several studies [14, 16, 24, 31–33]. High cholesterol may be a consequence of poor dietary habits, a sedentary lifestyle, and excessive alcohol consumption. The present finding, therefore, highlights the need to tailor primary prevention strategies towards reducing specific lifestyle behaviours that contribute to high LDL cholesterol and triglycerides among people with hypertension and/or diabetes. These predictors also go along with obesity—another predictor that was found to be associated with a high predicted risk of the composite outcome of heart failure or stroke. These findings are in keeping with what has been reported in other studies [15, 22, 27, 31]. A previous study from Ghana showed that only 16.8%. of adults with diabetes were on statins for risk reduction against MACE [34].

Moreover, prior diagnosis of heart attack was found to be highly predictive of the composite outcome. To the best of our knowledge however, this study is the first to specify the predictive impact of previous heart attack on the composite outcome of heart failure and stroke among persons with hypertension and diabetes in Ghana. This association has been reported in other studies elsewhere that examined heart failure and stroke as separate events [23, 35, 36]. In a very large prospective study of over 1.4 million individuals in Denmark, for instance, Sundbøll and colleagues confirmed heart attack as a risk factor for stroke, especially within the first year [37]. Given that coronary artery disease and ischemic stroke share common vascular risk factors, it is not surprising that previous heart attack was associated with incident stroke and heart failure. This finding particularly highlights the low rates of utilization of secondary prevention medications such as aspirin and statins in the public sector in many LMICs such as Ghana [34]. Our finding therefore has practical implications for intensive monitoring and management of persons with hypertension and diabetes who have a history of a heart attack.

Furthermore, the analysis showed that higher levels of glycated haemoglobin (HbA1c) at enrolment were associated with the composite outcome. Consistent with the present findings, previous studies have also concluded that prolonged hyperglycaemia is an important risk factor for heart failure or stroke [35, 38, 39]. Hyperglycaemia is thought to incite anaerobic metabolism, lactic acidosis, and production of free radicals, and thus directly affects vascular structure and function, which could lead to ischemic stroke [40, 41].

Some strengths and limitations that should however guide interpretations of the study findings are presented below. First, the study design was robust and therefore gives credence to the quality of data used for the analysis. Second, the assessment of exposures before outcomes also reduced temporal bias since it clearly defined temporality. The relatively large sample size used provided substantial statistical power for the analysis. Moreover, the use of LASSO was efficient as it can deal with overfitting and multicollinearity compared with other methods. Regarding study limitations, not all possible variables were measured at baseline. Therefore, other important predictors may have been missed. Future studies could investigate other variables including genetic biomarkers. Additionally, the LASSO regression was unable to include or exclude categorical variables in the output as whole entities but rather selected only informative levels within the variable due to the use of one hot encoding. Nonetheless, our study makes significant contribution to rapidly growing literature on stroke and heart failure incidence and prediction among risk groups.

CONCLUSION. The incidence rate of the composite outcome of heart failure and stroke is quite high among persons with hypertension and diabetes. However, males, past smokers, and unemployed people have significantly higher predicted risk of developing the adverse outcomes. In addition, previous diagnosis of a heart attack, high levels of triglycerides, and having both hypertension and T2D were highly predictive of heart failure or stroke incidence. The two models presented have appreciable discriminatory ability (c-index 0.79 and 0.74) although further validation is needed. The identified predictors could be informative for a more focused health education and counselling plan, and the monitoring of lipid profiles for at-risk persons including persons with a history of a heart attack.—

REFERENCES

1 Attaei MW, Khatib R, McKee M, et al. Availability and affordability of blood pressure-lowering medicines and the effect on blood pressure control in high-income, middle-income, and low-income countries: an analysis of the PURE study data. Lancet Public Health 2017; 2: e411–e419. **2** Javaroni V, Neves MF. Erectile Dysfunction and Hypertension: Impact on Cardiovascular Risk and Treatment. Int J Hypertens 2012; 2012: 627278. **3** Vos T, Lim SS, Abbafati C, et al. Global burden of 369 diseases and injuries in 204 countries and territories, 1990–2019: a systematic analysis for the Global Burden of Disease Study 2019. The Lancet 2020; 396: 1204–1222. **4** World Health Organization. Hypertension, https://www.who.int/news-room/fact-sheets/detail/hypertension (2021, accessed 2 August 2021). **5** Seid MA. Health-related quality of life and extent of self-care practice among heart failure patients in Ethiopia. Health Qual Life Outcomes 2020; 18: 27. **6** Tannor EK, Norman BR, Adusei KK, et al. Quality of life among patients with moderate to advanced chronic kidney disease in Ghana - a single centre study. BMC Nephrol 2019; 20: 122. **7** Upadhya B, Kitzman DW. Heart failure with preserved ejection fraction: New approaches to diagnosis and management. Clin Cardiol 2020; 43: 145–155. **8** Gallagher J, McDonald K, Ledwidge M, et al. Heart Failure in Sub-Saharan Africa. Card Fail Rev 2018; 4: 21–24. **9** Zannad F. Rising incidence of heart failure demands action. The Lancet 2018; 391: 518–519. **10** Lippi G, Sanchis-Gomar F. Global epidemiology and future trends of heart failure. AME Med J 2020; 5: 15–15. **11** Savarese G, Becher PM, Lund LH, et al. Global burden of heart failure: a comprehensive and updated review of epidemiology. Cardiovasc Res 2022; cvac013.**12** Bergsten TM, Nicholson A, Donnino R, et al. Predicting adults likely to develop heart failure using readily available clinical information. Prev Med 2020; 130: 105878. **13** Krishnamurthi RV, Ikeda T, Feigin VL. Global, Regional and Country-Specific Burden of Ischaemic Stroke, Intracerebral Haemorrhage and Subarachnoid Haemorrhage: A Systematic Analysis of the Global Burden of Disease Study 2017. Neuroepidemiology 2020; 54: 171–179. **14** Akinyemi RO, Owolabi MO, Ihara M, et al. Stroke, cerebrovascular diseases and vascular cognitive impairment in Africa. Brain Res Bull 2019; 145: 97–108. **15** Owolabi M, Olowoyo P, Popoola F, et al. The epidemiology of stroke in Africa: A systematic review of existing methods and new approaches. J Clin Hypertens 2018; 20: 47–55. **16** Sarfo FS, Mobula LM, Plange-Rhule J, et al. Incident stroke among Ghanaians with hypertension and diabetes: A multicenter, prospective cohort study. J Neurol Sci 2018; 395: 17–24. **17** Sarfo FS, Norman B, Appiah L, et al. Factors associated with incidence of stroke and heart failure among people living with HIV in Ghana: Evaluating Vascular Event Risk while on Long-Term Antiretroviral Suppressive Therapy (EVERLAST) Study. J Clin Hypertens 2021; 23: 1252–1259. **18** Sarfo FS, Mobula LM, Adade T, et al. Low blood pressure levels & incident stroke risk among elderly Ghanaians with hypertension. J Neurol Sci 2020; 413: 116770. **19** Institute for Health Metrics and Evaluation. GBD Compare | IHME Viz Hub, http://vizhub.healthdata.org/gbd-compare (2019, accessed 3 April 2022). **20** Brentnall AR, Cuzick J. Use of the concordance index for predictors of censored survival data. Stat Methods Med Res 2018; 27: 2359. **21** Alonso A, Barnes AE, Guest JL, et al. HIV Infection and Incidence of Cardiovascular Diseases: An Analysis of a Large Healthcare Database. J Am Heart Assoc 2019; 8: e012241. **22** Ntiyani N, Letamo G, Keetile M. Prevalence of and factors associated with hypertension, diabetes, stroke and heart attack multimorbidity in Botswana: Evidence from STEPS 2014 survey. PLOS ONE 2022; 17: e0265722. **23** Jenča D, Melenovský V, Stehlik J, et al. Heart failure after myocardial infarction: incidence and predictors. ESC Heart Fail 2021; 8: 222–237. **24** Tsao CW, Aday AW, Almarzooq ZI, et al. Heart Disease and Stroke Statistics—2022 Update: A Report From the American Heart Association. Circulation 2022; 145: e153–e639. **25** Elyamani R, Soulaymani A, Hami H. Epidemiology of Cardiovascular Diseases in Morocco: A Systematic Review. Rev Diabet Stud 2021; 17: 57–67. **26** Fekadu G, Chelkeba L, Kebede A. Risk factors, clinical presentations and predictors of stroke among adult patients admitted to stroke unit of Jimma university medical center, south west Ethiopia: prospective observational study. BMC Neurol 2019; 19: 187. **27** Alloubani A, Saleh A, Abdelhafiz I. Hypertension and diabetes mellitus as a predictive risk factors for stroke. Diabetes Metab Syndr Clin Res Rev 2018; 12: 577–584. **28** Fuchs FD, Whelton PK. High Blood Pressure and Cardiovascular Disease. Hypertension 2020; 75: 285–292. **29** Mefford MT, Goyal P, Howard G, et al. The association of hypertension, hypertension duration, and control with incident heart failure in black and white adults. J Clin Hypertens 2020; 22: 857–866. **30** Oh GC, Cho H-J. Blood pressure and heart failure. Clin Hypertens 2020; 26: 1. **31** Åberg ND, Adiels M, Lindgren M, et al. Diverging trends for onset of acute myocardial infarction, heart failure, stroke and mortality in young males: role of changes in obesity and fitness. J Intern Med 2021; 290: 373–385. **32** Biondi-Zoccai G, Peruzzi M, Frati G. Is Smoking Cessation the Best Intervention Ever to Prevent Heart Failure? J Am Coll Cardiol 2022; 79: 2306–2309. **33** Feodoroff M, Harjutsalo V, Forsblom C, et al. Dose-dependent effect of smoking on risk of coronary heart disease, heart failure and stroke in individuals with type 1 diabetes. Diabetologia 2018; 61: 2580–2589. **34** Sarfo FS, Ovbiagele B. Prevalence and predictors of statin utilization among patient populations at high vascular risk in Ghana. J Neurol Sci 2020; 414: 116838. **35** Mahaffey KW, Li J, Chang TI, et al. Independent predictors of heart failure in patients with type 2 diabetes and chronic kidney disease: modeling from the CREDENCE trial. Eur Heart J 2020; 41: ehaa946.1175. **36** Melendo-Viu M, Abu-Assi E, Manzano-Fernández S, et al. Incidence, prognosis and predictors of heart failure after acute myocardial infarction. REC CardioClinics 2020; 55: 8–14. **37** Sundbøll J, Horváth-Puhó E, Schmidt M, et al. Long-Term Risk of Stroke in Myocardial Infarction Survivors. Stroke 2016; 47: 1727–1733. **38** Mitsios JP, Ekinci EI, Mitsios GP, et al. Relationship Between Glycated Hemoglobin and Stroke Risk: A Systematic Review and Meta-Analysis. J Am Heart Assoc 2018; 7: e007858. **39** Shen Y, Shi L, Nauman E, et al. Association between Hemoglobin A1c and Stroke Risk in Patients with Type 2 Diabetes. J Stroke 2020; 22: 87. **40** Zhao W, Katzmarzyk PT, Horswell R, et al. Sex differences in the risk of stroke and HbA1c among diabetic patients. Diabetologia 2014; 57: 918–926. **41** Lindsberg PJ, Roine RO. Hyperglycemia in Acute Stroke. Stroke 2004; 35: 363–364.

AUTHORS

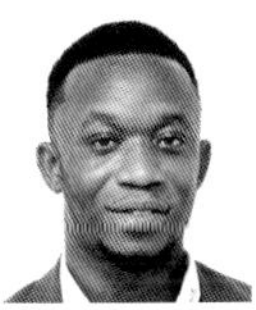

Robert Asampong
Corresponding author
Kumasi Centre for Collaborative Research in Tropical Medicine, Kumasi, Ghana
School of Public Health, Kwame Nkrumah University of Science and Technology (KNUST), Kumasi, Ghana
asampongrobbie@gmail.com

Yeetey Enuameh
School of Public Health, Kwame Nkrumah University of Science and Technology (KNUST), Kumasi, Ghana

Emmanuel Kweku Nakua
School of Public Health, Kwame Nkrumah University of Science and Technology (KNUST), Kumasi, Ghana

Gabriel Asare Okyere
Faculty of Physical and Computational Sciences, KNUST, Kumasi, Ghana

John Humphrey Amuasi
Kumasi Centre for Collaborative Research in Tropical Medicine, Kumasi, Ghana
School of Public Health, Kwame Nkrumah University of Science and Technology (KNUST), Kumasi, Ghana

Fred Stephen Sarfo
Komfo Anokye Teaching Hospital, Kumasi, Ghana
School of Medicine and Dentistry, KNUST, Kumasi, Ghana

#05 India
Experiences and perceptions of adolescents in menstrual health and hygiene in Dimapur, Nagaland

Sophia Loreni, Freya Brosterhus, Muriel Eckert
Co-Authors: Dr. Rhondemo Kikon, Prof. Timo Ulrichs, Gaby Feldmann, Janina Mitwalli, Tiajungla Aier

CHALLENGES IN MENSTRUAL HEALTH AND HYGIENE IN INDIA–SYNERGISTICALLY FINDING A WAY FORWARD THROUGH A COMMUNITY-BASED APPROACH. Menstruation has affected societies since the existence of mankind. It connects social interactions and health issues and has received increasing attention, especially in social media in the past few years. These public discussions often address topics such as the invisibility of menstruation in public as well as the access to menstrual hygiene products.

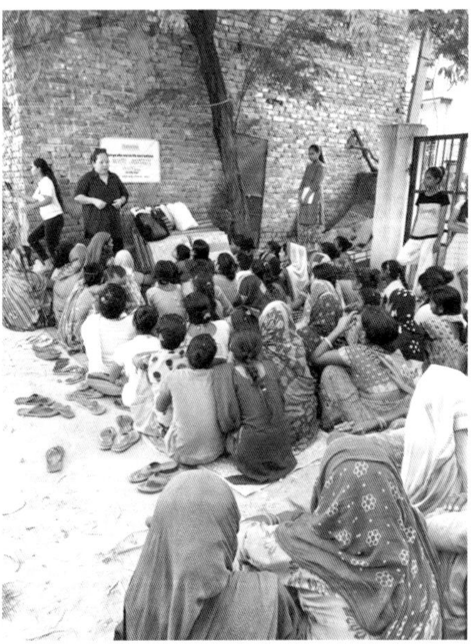

The topic has also been increasingly shed light on by researchers of various disciplines. A special focus is given on interlinkages between the handling of menstruation in society and the context of gender inequalities

In India, the government underlines challenges like e.g., a lacking supply of sanitary pads, as well as insufficient sanitary infrastructures. Within that, the handling of menstruation is linked with hygiene and reproductive health issues (cf. Das et al. 2015). To address these challenges, the Indian government published the Menstrual Hygiene Management National Guidelines in 2015 which highlight the normality of menstruation by referring to it as a biological and natural process. Apart from addressing the challenges to the sanitary infrastructure, the guidelines also link menstruation to stigma which affect the handling of menstrual health and hygiene management significantly (cf. Ministry of Drinking Water and Sanitation Government of India 2015, Ministry of Health and Family Welfare Government of India n.d.). Recent studies about the handling of menstruation in India demonstrate the linkage of gender related school absenteeism and the social stigma of menstruation (cf. van Eijk et al. 2015, Ganguli 2021).

To address circumstances of the handling of menstruation in rural areas, the Ministry of Health and Family Welfare, Government of India, launched the operational guidelines Menstrual Hygiene Scheme (MHS) in 2011 to promote menstrual hygiene among menstruating adolescents (between 10–19 years). MHS is linking low awareness and a lack of access to sanitary products to the neglect of menstrual hygiene. Myths and taboos surrounding menstruation are also understood as limiting menstruating adolescents from socializing and their access to schools, adding to the existing gender discrimination. Therefore schemes such as the MHS build on and strengthen interventions for adolescent girls by creating a forum for discussion on adolescent related issues such as early marriage, gender issues, nutrition, contraceptives, self-esteem, and negotiation skills, making available information and products related to improving menstrual hygiene (cf. National Rural Health Mission 2016).

Promoting adolescent health is an important part of reproductive and child health. To address challenges to adolescent health, the Adolescent Reproductive and Sexual Health (ARSH) and Adolescence Education Program (AEP) are core components of national health programs in India. Both these programs include a range of interventions for adolescent girls and boys who are in school and out of school.

IMPORTANCE OF VALUING LOCAL KNOWLEDGE AND EMPOWERING COMMUNITIES. Within approaches on the handling of menstruation, cultural and social norms as well as values related to subjects like gender, purity and cleanliness have a significant impact on menstrual experiences among adolescents (Gold-Watts and Hovdenak 2020: 8, 9). The importance of the cultural and social context becomes also clear by the critique of Indian activists and scholars who emphasize not to stigmatize local knowledge by simply applying concepts of hygiene and purity of the Global North. This may result in a "double victimization of women and girls, subjected not only to their own bodies, but also to the ignorance of their own families and communities" (2021: 198). Within this approach it is important to be aware of certain power relations regarding hierarchies of knowledge. As a consequence, valuing local knowledge and practices is necessary to better understand social and cultural dimensions of menstrual handling strategies (ebd., Bobel 2019: 27, McCarthy and Lahiri-Dutt 2020: 19, Lahiri-Dutt 2016: 10). It is important to take a look behind superficial challenges like a lack of supply of menstrual products. This more holistic approach might include the creation of a space for menstruators to share experiences, including the influence of social media as a source of information as well as raising awareness about menstruation among

#05 India
Experiences and perceptions of adolescents in menstrual health and hygiene in Dimapur, Nagaland

non-menstruators (Rawat et al. 2021: 3). The experiences and challenges around the handling of menstruation differ within local contexts in India.

For the reasons stated above, community-based approaches play a crucial role in applying national guidelines according to local circumstances as well as to adapt and develop new approaches according to the changing needs of menstruating adolescents.

The Community Health Initiative (CHI) in Nagaland, India for example, focuses on menstruating adolescents and women in Dimapur in the course of their project "Menstrual Initiative Nagaland". CHI's objective is to raise awareness about menstrual hygiene and the access to menstrual products within schools. The organization installed vending machines for sanitary napkins in schools, which work without electricity. Additionally it provided schools with incinerators to answer the disposal challenges of menstrual products in schools. Moreover, they conduct awareness and educational programmes in schools about menstrual hygiene. Since CHI focuses on livelihood as well, italso offer trainings to imprisoned women to sew their own cloth pads of old garments.

Another best practice of a community-based menstrual hygiene program was Pavna's unique model initiated by the Raigarh district in Chhattisgarh in 2021. The model functions on three principles: Access, Awareness, and Acceptance to bring a turnaround in behavior and usage patterns. The multiple government schemes ensured the channelization of resources for the program's functioning. The Pavna initiative encourages women from within the community to be agents of change. Therefore two women Self Help Groups (SHGs) were trained on sanitary production and entrepreneurship for an easy, cost-effective supply of sanitary pads in the community. Local volunteers also promoted menstrual hygiene through slogan writing, local folk songs, radio messaging, and street plays. In addition, school teachers, ASHA, and Anganwadi workers are also active participants in the initiative. Similarly, in fighting the taboo around menstruation, community leaders' and representatives' efforts were consistent during community meetings and one-to-one talks with elders to break myths and misconceptions surrounding the issue. Thus, for example, the initiative increased women's use of sanitary pads in the Raigarh district from 40 percent to 75 percent in just around one year, according to a study by the district's Women and Child Development department (cf. Singh et al. 2022).

CONCLUSION. Ultimately, menstruation is deeply intertwined with social and cultural norms and values. That's why challenges adolescents have to face during their menstruation have to be considered in a cultural and social context as well.

This emphasizes the necessity of local community-based approaches on one hand to recognize possible needs of adolescents in the context of social and cultural norms and values and on the other hand to apply approaches within local circumstances. To understand menstrual experiences in a deeper and more comprehensive sense and to avoid a double-victimization of menstruators, a holistic approach is necessary. This strategy includes factors like local concepts of body and hygiene and puts cultural backgrounds like religion into consideration.

ONGOING RESEARCH: MENSTRUAL EXPERIENCES AND PRACTICES OF ADOLESCENTS IN DIMAPUR, NAGALAND, INDIA. In Nagaland, India, only a rare number of studies and data addressing menstruation can be found. To contribute to the scientific data gap and to get to know possible challenges adolescents have to face during their menstruation in Nagaland, the authors conducted a qualitative research in the period October to December 2022. To avoid stigmatizing local knowledge the research is based on the approach of the grounded theory. The experiences of menstruating adolescents are put into center. The research seeks to gain an insight and deeper understanding of how adolescents handle their menstruation in their everyday life and which factors influence their menstrual handling and experiences significantly. In that matter education, circumstances in school, as well as structures of their daily life play a major role.

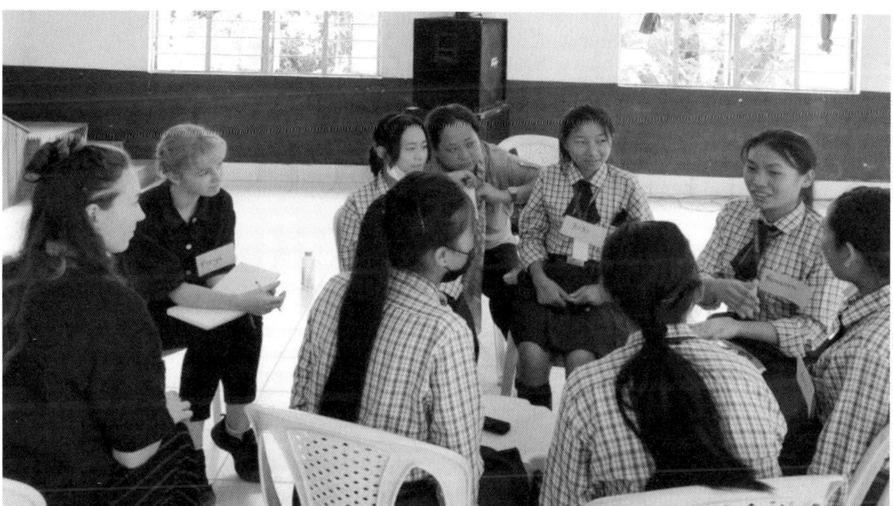

#05 India
Experiences and perceptions of adolescents in menstrual health and hygiene in Dimapur, Nagaland

The research project is taking place in both urban and rural areas of Dimapur in cooperation with the Community Health Initiative (CHI). In this interest, CHI and the Akkon University for Applied Human Sciences in Berlin co-initiated a research cooperation as part of the ASA (Arbeits- und Studienaufenthalte)-programme 2022. ASA is offered by Engagement Global and funded by the German Federal Ministry of Economic Cooperation and Development (BMZ). This collaborative research project is interested in gaining scientific data on individual experiences and practices as well as the social perceptions of menstruation in Nagaland. The different methods, such as group discussions and in-depth interviews with adolescents, as well as expert interviews, allow to get a profound insight into individual experiences and potential needs of adolescent girls.

Due to the short duration of three months and the focus only in the district of Dimapur, the research simply provides a starting point and can function as a basis for further research and action in the whole state of Nagaland. The data has been collected and is now in the analysis phase. The findings will be ready by spring 2023.—

REFERENCES

1 Bobel, C., 2019. The Managed Body: Developing Girls and Menstrual Health in the Global South, 1st ed. 2019. ed. Springer International Publishing: Imprint: Palgrave Macmillan, Cham. **2** Das, P., Baker, K.K., Dutta, A., Swain, T., Sahoo, S., Das, B.S., Panda, B., Nayak, A., Bara, M., Bilung, B., Mishra, P.R., Panigrahi, P., Cairncross, S., Torondel, B., 2015. Menstrual Hygiene Practices, WASH Access and the Risk of Urogenital Infection in Women from Odisha, India. PLoS ONE 10 (6), pp. 1–16.; **3** Ganguli, B., 2021. Menstrual Hygiene Management: Linking with Education and Development. ANTYAJAA: Indian Journal of Women and Social Change 6,pp. 47–60. **4** Gold-Watts, A., Hovdenak, M., Daniel, M., Gandhimathi, S., Sudha, R., Bastien, S., 2020. A qualitative study of adolescent girls' experiences of menarche and menstruation in rural Tamil Nadu, India. International Journal of Qualitative Studies on Health and Well-being 15 (1), pp. 1–14. **5** van Eijk, A.M., Sivakami, M., Thakkar, M.B., Bauman, A., Laserson, K.F., Coates, S., Phillips-Howard, P.A., 2016. Menstrual hygiene management among adolescent girls in India: a systematic review and meta-analysis. BMJ Open 6, pp. 1–12 **6** Lahiri-Dutt, K., 2014. Medicalising menstruation: a feminist critique of the political economy of menstrual hygiene management in South Asia. Gender, Place & Culture 22, pp. 1158–1176. **7** McCarthy, A., Lahiri-Dutt, K., 2020. Bleeding in Public? Rethinking Narratives of Menstrual Management from Delhi's Slums, in: Bobel, C., Winkler, I.T., Fahs, B., Hasson, K.A., Kissling, E.A., Roberts, T.-A. (Eds.), The Palgrave Handbook of Critical Menstruation Studies. Springer Singapore, Singapore, pp. 15–30. **8** McCarthy, A., Lahiri-Dutt, K., 2021. Producing knowledge of difference, producing different knowledge: Exploring the epistemic terrains of menstruation in India. Gender, Place & Culture 28, pp. 192–207. **9** Ministry of Drinking Water and Sanitation Government of India, GOI [WWW Document], 2015 URL https://jalshakti-ddws.gov.in/publication/menstrual-hygiene-management-national-guidelines-december-2015 (accessed 16.9.22). **10** Ministry of Health and Family Welfare Government of India, n.d. MENSTRUAL HEALTH IN INDIA: 1 AN UPDATE MENSTRUAL HEALTH IN INDIA: [WWW Document], n.d. URL https://www.studocu.com/in/document/dharmsinh-desai-university/mba/hiren-3-for-the-study-purpose/25951730 (accessed 8.9.22). **11** National Rural Health Mission, 2016. Operational guidelines on promotion of menstrual hygiene among adolescent girls (10–19 years) in rural areas URL https://nhm.gov.in/images/pdf/programmes/arsh/guidelines/MHS-operational-guidelines.pdf (accessed 12.12.22) **12** Rawat, M., Shields, A.N., Venetis, M.K., Seth, J., 2021. Women's Agentic Role in Enabling and Dismantling Menstrual Health Taboos in Northern India: A

Culture-Centred Approach. Health Communication, pp. 1–10. **13** Singh, B., Srivastava, R. and M. Ravi 2022. Pavna: A unique community-based menstrual hygiene programm. In Observer Research Observation. URL https://www.orfonline.org/expert-speak/pavna-a-unique-community-based-menstrual-hygiene-programme/ (accessed 29.12.2022)

AUTHORS

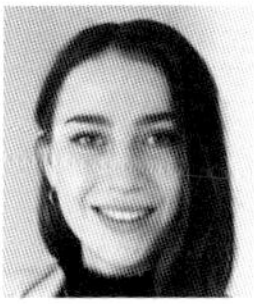

Muriel Eckert
B.A. International Emergency and Disaster Relief | Akkon University for Human Sciences
E-mail: muriel-eckert@web.de | Tel. +4915122847831

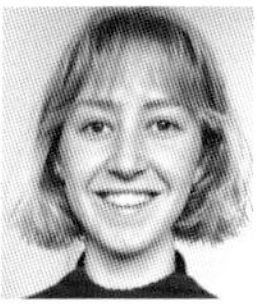

Freya Brosterhus
M.A Social and Cultural Anthropology | Free University Berlin
E-mail: freya.brosterhus@web.de | Tel. +49 15788253683

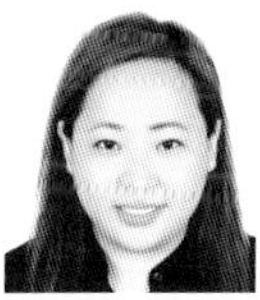

Sophia Loreni (BA, LLB)
Advisor Community Health Initiative
E-mail: loreni.sophia@gmail.com | Tel. +91-8259062117

FURTHER INFORMATION ABOUT THE COMMUNITY-BASED INITIATIVE

Community Health Initiative, Nagaland, India:
Address: Duncan Bosti, House House No 55, 1st Floor Pincode: 797112, Nagaland, India
E-mail: adm@chi.org.in | Tel. +91-9863347778 | Website: www.chi.org.in

#06.1 Indonesia
Public Health and Climate Change: An Indonesian Perspective
Hannah Becker

With 17,500 islands, Indonesia is the largest archipelago in the world. Administratively, Indonesia consists of 34 provinces, including the special capital region of Jakarta. Provinces consist of districts and communes, which are divided into sub-districts, which in turn are divided into administrative villages. With more than 700 different groups, the Indonesian population is ethnically, culturally and linguistically very diverse (cf. WHO 2017). Indonesia is the fourth most populous country with nearly 273.5 million people in 2020, which is forecast to reach 295 million in 2030 (cf. UN 2021). The population of Indonesia has been subject to demographic change for several years. Annual population growth has declined from 1.8% in 1990 to 1.2% in 2015. The proportion of elderly population is increasing (5.1% of the population is 65 years or older) (cf. The World Bank 2020). Urbanization in Indonesia is among the fastest in Asia: between 2010 and 2015, the urban population grew at an average rate of 2.7% per year, with more than half of the population living in cities in 2015 (ebd. 2020). In 2018, there were around 4.3 doctors for every 10,000 inhabitants (cf. UN 2021).

The Universal Health Coverage Index increased from 30.0 in 2000 to 57.0 in 2017 (cf. UN 2021). On January 1, 2014, Indonesia began sweeping health insurance reforms as part of its efforts to achieve Universal Health Coverage (UHC). Health insurance should gradually cover 257.5 million people by 2019 (cf. WHO 2019). Although around one in ten Indonesians lives below the poverty line, 175 million people, almost a third of the population, have health insurance (cf. GIZ 2017). Net disbursements of total ODA received for medical research in 2018 were $55.2 million in the healthcare sector (cf. GIZ 2017)(cf. BMZ 2021). Indicators of general health in Indonesia have improved significantly, with life expectancy at birth increasing from 66.3 years in 2000 to 69.1 years in 2015 (cf. UN 2021). Another achievement is lower infant and child mortality. The rate fell from 187,172.0 in 2000 to 102,086.0 in 2018. The under-five mortality rate fell from 52.4 deaths per 1,000 live births in 2000 to 25.0 deaths per 1,000 live births in 2018 (cf. UN 2021). Less progress has been made in improving maternal mortality and malnutrition. The rate fell from 272.0 per 100,000 live births in 2000 to 177.0 per 100,000 live births in 2017 (cf. UN 2021). Currently, maternal, newborn and child health are among the top health priorities in Indonesia. To this end, Indonesia has made a variety of national and global commitments, such as expanding universal coverage of maternal health services and strengthening childhood immunization programs, as well as the SDG´s in Maternal, Newborn and Child Health of the Millenniums -Advancing the development goals of the United Nations (cf. Davis 2015).

Patterns in disease epidemiology in Indonesia indicate an increasingly complex health situation. While communicable diseases remain a significant problem, noncommunicable diseases are becoming more prevalent. Nevertheless, the proportion of the target population with access to a second-dose vaccine containing measles (MCV2) rose from 21.0% in 2003 to 67.0% in 2018 (cf. UN 2021). In 2015, four of the top 10 causes of premature death were noncommunicable diseases, five were communicable, maternal, neonatal and diet-related diseases, and one was injuries (cf. UN 2021) Tropical diseases also pose a major challenge, particularly among the poorer population. The most widespread neglected tropical diseases include lymphatic filariasis and bacterial infections such as yaws and leptospirosis (cf. Cbm o.J.). The number of people requiring interventions against neglected tropical diseases was 100,847,287.0 in 2018 (cf. UN 2021).

Inequalities between geographic areas and income levels are significant and pose a major challenge to health systems. Demographic and epidemiological changes have impacted the burden of disease: disability-adjusted life years (DALYs) due to cerebrovascular disease, cardiovascular disease, diabetes and lung cancer are increased by 80% or more between 1990 and 2010. The central government had committed to introducing Universal Health Coverage (UHC) by 2019, as projected in the Jaminan Kesehatan Nasional (JKN) or National Health Insurance Program Road Map, 2012–2019 (cf. Dartanto 2017). The current COVID situation is that 56% of the population is fully vaccinated and 15% partially vaccinated. A total of 5.96 million cases have been recorded, of which 154,000 were fatal (Cf. Dartanto 2017).

Thematically, climate change, air pollution, food security, water management or even antibiotic resistance can serve as examples to show the connections between humans and nature and their influence on health.

For Indonesia, in concrete figures, in 2016 the death rate attributable to air pollution was 51.0 deaths per 1,000 people. The mortality rate, which is partly due to unclean water, was 7.1 deaths per 1000 inhabitants in 2016 (cf. O.V. 2016). Other impacts of climate change include increased risk of water-borne and vector-borne diseases, rising sea levels and resulting flooding. Due to increased temperatures, drought cycles are also a challenge for food production and thus for the food security of the population (cf. O.V. 2016).

This is linked to the interaction of the structures of the health system such as universities, hospitals and professionals, their function, how they relate to each other and how this develops over time, i.e. which process they go through. Medical care is a crucial point here. The example of mortality rates from climate-related causes affecting the entire population makes it clear how important it is to create a health system in which all citizens are covered. The world's largest contributory statutory health insurance system was introduced in 2014 as a result of an initiative by the Indonesian government with the support of the GIZ. Around 90 million Indonesians living on the poverty line and a total of around two thirds of the population are protected as a result. The health system structures in rural areas that have been hit even harder by climate disasters were also expanded as part of this initiative (cf. GIZ 2017).

In the case of the chosen example of climate change, this is a long-term problem and accordingly cannot be solved with short-term strategies, but permanent initiatives of the same kind that change the structure are required here.

Both the MDGs and the SDGs can be classified in the connection between economic performance, ecology, politics and, of course, social issues. The impact of environmental influences on population health is a good example of this. The ecological factors influence the social area through damage to health, which must be counteracted by political and economic measures. Thus, through this one problem, all areas are involved and in interaction with each other.

In order to be able to guarantee the best possible population health, politicians must look at the health sector from their point of view and include the view of the population as perceived space in concepts. Also, the field of health has to be related to others, for example when it comes to financing, it is not insignificant for health to enable good education in order to be able to train health professionals.

Health-influencing factors are often so far-reaching that they are developed from local approaches through regional, national and international to global discussions. Climate change is being tackled at all levels to protect people's health. Nationally, Indonesia combats existing damage, while globally SDG´s prevent further harm.

The example of global warming shows that in order to reduce or prevent harmful consequences and to counteract the current development, this problem cannot only be tackled unilaterally. This requires cooperation within the areas of a country, as well as cooperation of this country globally with other countries. Based on this consideration, the state of public health can be traced back to a large extent to climate catastrophes and other climate change impacts listed above. Floods in particular have been devastating since Indonesia consists of a large number of islands.

Adaption is an important aspect of climate change. The World Health Organisation (WHO) established an adaption policy for climate change that was adopted by the Government of Indonesia (GOI) and comprises the following points: Health development, evidence and information, delivers and partnership, strengthened health systems. The National Program of Adaptation an Mitigation aims to build environmental health capacity building, infectious disease surveillance, health action in emergencies, safe drinking water, integrated vector management and healthy public policy.

CONCLUSION AND RECOMMENDATION. Despite the fact that climate change is a worldwide concern, Indonesia as an archipelagic country has special challenges. These include the vulnerability of residents of tiny islands and coastal regions to sea level rise; the spread of serious mosquito-borne illnesses, including malaria and dengue fever, into regions where immunity is low; and the rise in water-borne illnesses and malnutrition. Although existing efforts and coping measures, it is still essential to develop effective multi sectoral public health strategies for Indonesia`s climate change.—

REFERENCES

Bundesministerium für wirtschaftliche Zusammenarbeit und Entwicklung (2021): Politisches Schwergewicht in Südostasien | https://www.bmz.de/de/laender/indonesien • Cbm (o.J.): Vernachlässigte Tropenkrankheiten https://www.cbm.de/informieren/vermeidbare-behinderungen/sehbehinderungen/vernachlaessigte-tropenkrankheiten.html • Dartanto, Teguh (2017): Universal Health Coverage in Indonesia | https://www.imf.org/-/media/Files/News/Seminars/2A2_Presenter_Dartanto.ashx • Davis, Ben (2015): Indonesias`s Millennium Development Goal report card | https://www.insideindonesia.org/indonesia-s-millennium-development-goal-report-card • Fögele, Janis (2016). Adaption der Geographischen Basiskonzepte https://edoc.hu-berlin.de/bitstream/handle/18452/23690/ZGD-46-1-Foegele.pdf;jsessionid=193262F0BFC2086BB9E0107A33529B3B?sequence=3 • GIZ (Deutsche Gesellschaft für Internationale Zusammenarbeit)(2017): Indonesien: Eine Krankenversicherung für alle | https://www.giz.de/de/mediathek/55430.html • GIZ (2017): Indonesien: Eine Krankenversicherung für alle| https://www.giz.de/de/mediathek/55430.html • GOI (2022): National Adaption Plan 2022 | https://lcdi-indonesia.id/wp-content/uploads/2020/05/Executive-Summary-NAP.pdf) • Our World in data (2022): Share of people vaccinated against COVID-19, March 20, 2022 | https://ourworldindata.org/covid-vaccinations?country=IDN • The World Bank (2020): Indonesien | https://datacommons.org/place/country/IDN?utm_medium=explore&mprop=count&popt=Person&hl=de • United Nations (2021). SDG Country Profile Indonesia | https://unstats.un.org/sdgs/dataportal/countryprofiles/IDN#goal-3 • WHO (2017): The Republic of Indonesia Health System Review https://apps.who.int/iris/bitstream/handle/10665/254716/9789290225164-eng.pdf • WHO (2019): Primary Health Care on the Road to Universal Health Coverage | https://www.who.int/docs/default-source/documents/2019-uhc-report.pdf • WHO (2022): W.Climate Change • https://www.who.int/health-topics/climate-change#tab=tab_1 • O.V. (2016): Highlighting the unique link between climate change and health https://unfccc.int/news/human-health-needs-a-healthy-planet

AUTHOR

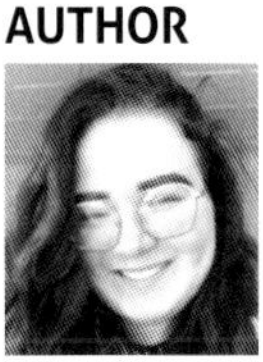

Hannah Becker
Student International Emergency and Disaster Relief (4th semester)
Akkon Hochschule für Humanwissenschaften,
Research Assistant IRIA

#06.2 Indonesia
Smoking behavior among university students in Germany and Indonesia: a comparative study

Hani Nasr, Timo Ulrichs, Nida Amalia, Sri Sunarti, Kresna Febriyanto, Erliga Nur Hikmah, Gandi Puad Pratama, Gaby Feldmann, Ghozali

BACKGROUND & OBJECTIVE. Tobacco usage is a leading cause of morbidity and mortality worldwide. This study aims to analyze health awareness and attitudes towards smoking among university students in Indonesia and Germany and their association with smoking behavior.

METHODS. This is a cross-sectional analysis of data collected using pretested structured questionnaire from the university students in Germany and Indonesia.

RESULTS. Most students (87%) are aware of major health risk related to smoking with insignificant difference between German and Indonesian contexts. The majority (95%) of respondents presented an attitude against smoking with an insignificant difference between both contexts. Only 13% of students were current smokers with a significant difference between the two contexts. Eighty-three percent (83%) reported presence of someone in the surroundings such as family members, friend or colleague who smokes with higher rate in Germany. In regression analysis there was a positive association between male sex and smoking behavior (OR, 1.8; 95%CI, 1–3.1). High academic level had a negative association with smoking behavior in bivariable analysis (OR, 0.3; 95%CI, 0.2–0.6). On bivariable analysis there was a negative association between good knowledge and smoking behavior (OR, 0.6; 95 0.33–1). Students with attitude proponent for smoking had positive association with smoking behavior in multiple regression model (OR, 4; 95%CI, 1.7–9.1). Presence of someone in the surrounding environment who smokes such as family members and friends was positively associated with smoking behavior (OR, 4.4; 95_%CI, 1.34–14.56). There was no significant association between different kinds of advertisements and smoking behavior. Receiving any kind of promotions was strongly associated with smoking behavior (OR, 2.3; 95%CI, 1.1–4.5). The effect of different factors on smoking behavior was the same in both German and Indonesian contexts.

CONCLUSION. There are several factors determining smoking behavior among university students including social factors and awareness level about potential health risks. Successful smoking prevention programs should consider the social environment's influence on the start and maintenance of smoking behavior, including the effect of parents, peers, and friends. Effective anti-smoking campaigns should intentionally target people's beliefs and attitudes and aim to persuade people and change their behavior, rather than simply delivering information. Anti-smoking policies should take into account the effect of tobacco advertisements and promotional activities.

KEYWORDS. Tobacco; Smoking; Germany; Indonesia; Awareness; Attitude

INTRODUCTION. Tobacco usage is a leading cause of chronic diseases such as cardiovascular disease and lung cancer and the single most preventable cause of death and disease[1]. According to Global Burden of Disease Study, there were 1.14 billion current smokers worldwide, who used 7.41 trillion cigarette-equivalents of tobacco. Smoking tobacco usage was also the greatest cause of mortality among males, accounting for 7.69 million deaths and 200 million disability-adjusted life-years globally. Current smokers accounted for 6.68 million (86.9%) of the 7.69 million deaths caused by tobacco use. China, India, Indonesia, the United States, Russia, Bangladesh, Japan, Turkey, Vietnam, and the Philippines were the ten nations with the most tobacco smokers in 2019[2].

In comparison to other Western and Northern European countries, Germany has a very high tobacco usage rate. Current tobacco use was found to be 28.3 percent in the entire survey population and 11.9 percent among those under the age of 18[3]. However, this figure is much better than the conditions in 1998, where the total prevalence of smoking was 30.2%. According to statistics from the Socio-Economic Panel (SOEP), a behavioral change among younger people, drove the decline in smoking prevalence and average cigarette use[4]. Some studies showed that school programs emphasizing the development of abilities to recognize and resist negative influences, extensive use of media and technological equipment, and health warnings have all proven to be beneficial in lowering tobacco use[5].

In Indonesia, smokers account for 40.3 percent of the population which place Indonesia is one of the countries with the highest prevalence of smokers in the world[6]. Prevalence of male and female smokers based on age group is 15–24 (51.7%: 0.1%), 25–44 (73.3%: 1.7%), 45–64 (72.4%: 5.8%) and 65+ (61.2%: 6.7%). According to the national statistics IN 2011, 89.3 percent of teenagers in Indonesia saw cigarette advertisements on billboards, 76.6 percent in magazines or newspapers, and 7.7% received free cigarettes. In stores where cigarettes are sold, 8 out of 10 adults thought cigarette advertisements[7]. The anti-smoking advertisement, on the other hand, had a far lower rating. Only 4 out of 10 adults perceived anti-tobacco advertising with television or radio. When contrasted pro-smoking material, this indicates that we have a large number of people who have been exposed to cigarette advertising. The most recent anti-smoking campaign in Indonesia has been broadcasted on television since June 2014[8].

The role of the media in promoting and reducing tobacco Use is significant. Anti-tobacco media campaigns are effective in reduceing smoking among youth and adults according to a report released in June 2008 by the National Cancer Institute (NCI), and particularly advertisements that evoke strong emotions have the most impact on viewers, and youth also react positively to anti-tobacco advertisements[9]. Based on a study published in June 2006, an increased exposure to state sponsored anti-tobacco media campaigns increase smoking cessation rates, even after controlling for other factors that may affect smoking cessation. Researchers found in particular that the quit rate among adult smokers increased by about ten percent in communities exposed to higher levels of states anti-tobacco advertising[10].

Knowledge and attitude towards smoking is well established in the literature. According to a cross/sectional study conducted in Bangalore, India, knowledge of the risks of smoking was high among the study population, and the vast majority of participants had negative attitude towards smoking[11]. Regarding the effect of knowledge and attitude on smoking behavior, a study conducted in USA found that knowledge and attitude are associated with smoking behavior. The study noted that the majority of smokers have low levels of health knowledge, suggesting that if health literacy were raised nationally, smoking rates would decrease[12]. Comparatively to respondents with higher attitude scores, the researchers found also, those with lower attitude scores were more likely to smoke cigarettes. This suggests that attitude has a big impact on quitting smoking[12, 13].

Several studies found that age, sex, and social factors were predictors of smoking behavior. The mother's educational level, the family's income, the presence of a smoker in the household, and the male gender are all significant risk factors for students' smoking behavior[14–18].

Young people develop nicotine dependence faster than adults do; therefore, it is crucial to start awareness interventions on young adults before they start smoking[19, 20]. This study is part of a joint project between Akkon University for Applied Human Sciences (Akkon) and Universitas Muhammadiyah Kalimantan Timur (UMKT), Indonesia aims to analyze health awareness and attitudes toward smoking among university students in Germany and Indonesia and their association with smoking behavior.

METHODS.

Study design, setting and sampling

This is a cross-sectional study. It was conducted in two universities in both East Kalimantan, Indonesia, and Berlin, Germany. After cluster sampling, 682 students were selected and interviewed through pretested questionnaire.

The main outcome was smoking status according to international definition [21].

Statistical analysis

Data were imported from an Excel spreadsheet and then analyzed using STATA 17.0 version.

RESULTS.

Sociodemographic characteristics

The socio-demographic characteristics of the study population are shown in Table 1. The age of the respondents ranged between 17 to 55 years with a mean age of 21 years (sd=4.8). Most respondents were below age of 20 (56.6%). There was female sex predominance among participants (73.6%). There was a significant difference in mean age between Germany and Indonesia with mean of 31& 20 years respectively (p<0.001). Female sex predominance was higher among Indonesian students with 79% of participants were female in comparison to only 35% among German.

Variable		Total (n=682) n(%)	Germany (DE) (n=85) n(%)	Indonesia (ID) (n=597) n(%)	P value*
Age	Age in years	21.5(4.9)¹	31.8(7.8)¹	20(1.15)¹	<0.001+
	Age≤ 20	385(56.6)	2(2.35)	383(64.37)	<0.001**
	Age> 20	295(43.38)	83(97.65)	212(35.63)	
Gender	Female	502(73.6)	30(35.3)	472(79)	<0.001**
	Male	180(26.39)	55(64.71)	125(20.94)	
Academic level	Bachelor	86(13.21)	81(95.29)	5(0.88)	<0.001**
	Master	565(86.79)	4(4.71)	561(99.12)	

* X^2 test for the difference in PR; ¹ mean (SD); ** statistically significant; + ttest of means

Table 1. Sociodemographic characteristics of the stude population (n=682): DE vs ID

Variable		Total (n=682) n(%)	DE (n=85) n(%)	ID (n=597) n(%)	P value*
Knowledge on risks of smoking	Good	594(87.10)	70(82.35)	524(87.77)	0.16
Attitude towards smoking	Opponent	647(94.87)	79(92.94)	568(95.14)	0.39
Smoking status	Non-smoker	510(74.78)	47(55.29)	463(77.55)	<0.001**
	Ex-smoker	81(11.88)	16(18.82)	65(10.89)	<0.001**
	Current smoker	91(13.34)	22(25.88)	69(11.56)	<0.001**
Current Smoking behavior	Yes	91(13.34)	22(25.88)	69(11.56)	<0.001**

* X^2 test; ** statistically significant

Table 2. Knowledge, attitude and smoking behavior among study participants

Knowledge, attitude and smoking behavior characteristics

Knowledge, attitude and smoking behavior characteristics of participants are summarized in table 2.

Eighty-seven percent (87%) of students had good knowledge score on smoking risks with insignificant difference between German and Indonesian students. The vast majority of respondents presented attitude against smoking (95%) with an insignificant difference between German and Indonesian contexts. Only 13% of students were current smokers with a significant difference between German and Indonesian students. One in four German students (26%) smokes compared to only 11% of Indonesian students.

Smoking practices, habits, reasons and other smoking characteristics

Smoking practices, habits, reasons and other smoking characteristics are presented in table 3. The majority of respondents reported presence of someone in the surroundings who smokes (84%), with borderline significant difference between German and Indonesian students; higher among German (p=0.07). Smoking friends were the main ones (77%) followed by parents and siblings (45% & 42% respectively). Smoking parents, siblings and friends were higher among Indonesian students (p, 0.002; <0.001; 0.007 respectively) while smoking colleagues and university members were higher among German students (p<0.001).

Forty percent (40%) smoke only during stress with an insignificant difference between German and Indonesian students. Around 40% of students smoke on a daily basis with significant difference between students of Germany and Indonesia where the number is higher among German (72%, p<0.001). Cigarettes was the most common type among participants (53%) with significantly higher percentage among German students (77%, p=0.01). According to respondents, the main reason for non-smoking was health aspect (82%) with significantly higher percentage

Variable		Total (n=682) n(%)	DE (n=85) n(%)	ID (n=597) n(%)	P value*
Someone in the Social environment is smoking	Yes (overall)	572(83.87)	77(90.59)	495(82.91)	0.07[δ]
	Parents	259(45.12)	22(28.57)	237(47.69)	0.002**
	Siblings	241(41.99)	14(18.18)	227(45.67)	<0.001**
	Friends	442(77)	50(64.94)	392(78.87)	0.007**
	Partner	66(11.50)	8(10.39)	58(11.67)	0.74
	Colleagues	132(23)	64(83.12)	68(13.68)	<0.001**
	University staff member	38(6.62)	14(18.18)	24(4.83)	<0.001**
Smoking habits *(total = 91, DE = 22, ID = 69)*	Daily	36(39.56)	16(72.73)	20(28.99)	<0.001**
	Evening after work	12(13.19)	5(22.73)		0.12
	Weekend	2(2.20)	0	2(3)	0.41
	When socializing	33(36.26)	40(40.91)	24(34.78)	0.60
	During stress	37(40.66)	12(54.55)	25(36.23)	0.12
	Others	24(26.37)	4(18.18)	20(28.99)	0.31
Smoking types *(total = 95, DE = 22, ID = 73)*	Cigarettes	51(53.68)	17(77.27)	34(46.58)	0.01**
	Pipes	5(5.26)	2(9)	3(4.11)	0.35
	Shisha	4(4.21)	1(4.55)	3(4.11)	0.92
	e-cigarettes	32(33.68)	6(27.27)	26(35.62)	0.46
	Others	19(20)	1(4.55)	18(24.66)	0.04**
Reason for non-smoking *(total = 89, DE = 17, ID = 72)*	Health	75(84.27)	17(100)	58(80.56)	0.04**
	Cost	40(45)	7(41.18)	33(45.83)	0.72
	Environment	31(34.83)	4(23.53)	27(37.5)	0.27
	Taste	15(16.85)	8(47)	7(9.72)	<0.001**
	Lack of benefit	41(46)	3(17.65)	38(52.78)	0.009**
Smoking reasons *(total = 87, DE = 22, ID = 65)*	Habit	43(49.43)	18(81.82)	25(38.46)	<0.001**
	Addiction	27(31)	15(68.18)	12(18.46)	<0.001**
	Social environment	32(36.78)	3(13.64)	29(44.62)	0.009**
	Stress	38(43.68)	14(63.64)	24(36.92)	0.02**
	Popularity	1(1.15)	0	1(1.54)	0.55
	Socialization	29(33.33)	10(45.45)	19(29.23)	0.16
Try stop *(total = 101, DE = 22, ID= 79)*	Yes	72(71.29)	16(72.73)	56(70.89)	0.86
Cessation means *(total = 84, DE = 17, ID = 67)*	NRT[1]	18(21.43)	3(17.65)	15(22.39)	0.67
	Drug therapy	3(3.57)	0	3(4.48)	0.37
	Counselling	12(14.29)	1(5.88)	11(16.42)	0.26
	Behavioral therapy	17(20.24)	0	17(25.37)	0.02**
	Nothing	41(48.81)	10(58.82)	31(46.27)	0.35

X^2 test; ** statistically significant; [δ]borderline significant

Table 3. Smoking practicies, habits, reasons and cessation

among German (p=0.04). other reasons were cost (45%), environment (35%), taste (17%) and lack of benefit (46%). Habitual smoking was the main reason of smoking (49.4%). Other reasons were addiction (31%), social environment (37%), stress (43.7%), popularity (1%) and socialization (33.3%). Habitual smoking, addiction and stress were significantly higher among German (p<0.001, p<0.001& p=0.02 respectively), while social environment was higher among Indonesian (p=0.009).

Variable		Total (n=682) n(%)	DE (n=85) n(%)	ID (n=597) n(%)	P value*
Exposure to Ads in the last 30 days (total = 676, DE = 84, ID = [illegible])	Yes	449 (66.42)	39(46.43)	110(69.26)	<0.001**
Exposure to ads	On clothes	114(16.72)	13(15.29)	101(16.92)	0.7
	Outdoor	423(62)	35(41.18)	388(65)	<0.001**
	Shopping mall	302(44.28)	10(11.76)	292(48.91)	<0.001**
	TV	348(51)	4(4.7)	344(57.6)	<0.001**
	Social media	223(32.7)	8(9.41)	215(36)	<0.001**
Location of ads (total = 452, DE = 39, ID = 413)	Public area	284(62.83)	30(76.92)	254(61.5)	0.05**
	shop	246(54.42)	20(51.28)	226(54.72)	0.68
	Poster/bill board	312(69)	25(64.1)	287(69.49)	0.48
	Others	27(5.97)	3(7.69)	24(5.81)	0.63
Receiving promotion		73(10.7)	3(3.53)	70(11.73)	0.02**

* X^2 test; ** statistically significant

Table 4. Exposure to tobacco advertising and promotion

Smoking advertisements (ads) and promotion

Smoking advertisements and promotion is presented in table 4. Almost two third of respondents (66%) reported exposure to advertisements within 30 days prior to the survey. Higher percentage observed among Indonesian students (p<0.001).

FACTORS ASSOCIATED WITH SMOKING BEHAVIOR

Bivariable analysis

Table 5 shows the bivariable associations between several independent factors and smoking behavior. Students with age above 20 years had higher odd of being smokers with borderline significance (OR, 1.5; 95%CI, 0.99–2.41; p=0.05). There was a strong positive statistically significant association between male sex and smoking behavior (OR, 3.68; 95%CI, 2.3–5.9; p<0.001). High academic level had a strong negative association with smoking behavior (OR, 0.3; 95%CI, 0.2–0.6, p<0.001). Being from Germany was positively associated with smoking behavior (OR, 2.7; 95%CI, 1.5–4.6; p<0.001). Although the close to borderline statistical significance there was negative association between good knowledge and smoking behavior (OR, 0.59; 95% CI, 0.33–1; p=0.07). Students with attitude proponent for smoking had statistically significant strong positive association with smoking behavior (OR, 9.5; 95%CI, 4.53–19.85; p<0.001). Presence of someone in the surrounding environment who smokes such as family member and friends was strongly positively associated with smoking behavior (OR, 4.75; 95%CI, 1.69–13.35; p=0.001). Specifying the surroundings into different social categories showed that only smoking colleague and university member have positive statistically

#06.2 Indonesia
Smoking behavior among university students in Germany and Indonesia: a comparative study

Variable	Odd ratio OR(95% CI)	P value*
Age >20	1.5(0.99-2.41)	0.05**
Sex (male)	3.7(2.3-5.9)	<0.001**
Academic level(master)	0.3(0.2 - 0.6)	<0.001**
Country (Germany)	2.7(1.5 - 4.6)	<0.001**
Knowledge (good)	0.59(0.33-1)	0.07'
Attitude (proponent)	9.5(4.53-19.85)	<0.001**
Social environment	4.75(1.69-13.35)	0.001**
Smoking parents	1.2(0.77- 1.93)	0.38
Smoking siblings	1.3(0.81- 2)	0.29
Smoking friends	0.86(0.51- 1.46)	0.58
Smoking partner	1.4(0.7- 2.8)	0.27
Smoking colleague	3 (1.87- 4.98)	<0.001**
Smoking university member	2 (0.99- 4.6)	0.04**
Exposure to ads in general	0.8(0.5 - 1.3)	0.3
Ads on clothes	1.4(0.8- 2.4)	0.25
Ads on billboard and outdoor	1.14(0.7- 1.8)	0.5
Ads in shopping mall	0.8 (0.5 - 1.2)	0.3
Ads on tv	0.7 (0.5 - 1.2)	0.2
Ads on social media	0.7(0.4 - 1.2)	0.16
Receiving at least one kind of promotion	4.6 (2.6 – 8)	<0.001**

χ^2 test; ** statistical significant; ' close to the significance level

Table 5. Bicariable associations between smoking behavior and other variables

significant association with smoking behavior (OR, 3; 95%CI, 1.87–4.98; p<0.001) and (OR,2; 95%CI, 0.99–4.6; p=0.04) respectively. Receiving any kind of promotions was strongly associated with smoking behavior (OR, 4.6; 95%CI, 2.6 – 8; p<0.001).

Multivariate analysis

Multivariable analysis has been performed only for those with enough or borderline evidence of association with the outcome variable, smoking behavior such as sex, academic level, attitude and promotion. Crude and adjusted odd ratios are presented in table 6.

Results of the logistic regression model showed that male sex, proponent attitude, social environment, and receiving promotion remained a significant predictors and risk factors for smoking behavior (ORs, 1.8, 4, 4.4, and 2.3 respectively). Although the knowledge lost its significant effect,

Variable	Crude OR OR(95% CI, p)*	Adjusted OR aOR (95% CI, p)**
Age>20	1.5 (0.99-2.41, p=0.5)	-
Male sex	3.7(2.3-5.9, p<0.001)	1.8(1-3.1, p=0.05)
Academic level (master)	0.3(0.2 - 0.6, p<0.001)	-
Country (Germany)	2.7(1.5 - 4.6, p<0.001)	
Good Knowledge	0.6(0.33-1, p= 0.07)	-
Proponent Attitude	9.5(4.53-19.85, p<0.001)	4(1.7 – 9.1, p=0.001)
Someone smoking in the surroundings	4.75(1.69-13.35, p=0.001)	4.4(1.34 – 14.56, p=0.01)
Receiving promotion	4.6 (2.6 – 8, p<0.001)	2.3(1.1 – 4.5, p=0.02)

OR, odd ratio; CI, confidence interval; * chi square test; ** Wald test;

Table 6. Multivariate analysis of associations between smoking behavior and other characteristics

the attitude was strong factor that can influence the smoking behavior.

The effect of different factors on smoking behavior was the same in both populations.

DISCUSSION. Tobacco use is a major health concern worldwide[1]. Young people, such as university students, require fewer smokes than adults do in order to become nicotine dependent, and when they start smoking, it will be exceedingly tough for them to stop, and they will keep smoking far into adulthood. Therefore, it is essential to begin education and awareness campaigns for young adults before they start smoking [19, 20]. A few studies have explored students' knowledge and attitudes toward smoking in the context of Indonesia and Germany. This study examines health knowledge, smoking attitudes, and smoking behavior among university students in Indonesia and Germany in order to predict the need and effectiveness of anti-smoking programs.

In the present study, most students were able to correctly identify the risks of smoking (87%). This is comparable with a study on knowledge, attitude and practice of cigarette smoking among students in Indonesia, the majority of students, were aware that smoking cigarettes has negative health effects [13]. Likewise another study in India found that 94% of respondents believed that smoking is definitely harmful to our health [11]. According to the current study 95% of respondents presented attitude against smoking, which agree with similar findings of a study in India [11]. The prevalence of smoking was 13%, which is relatively low in compare to similar studies on the prevalence of smoking among university students in Yemen and Malaysia where almost 30% of students were smokers [14, 22]. This could also be explained by the underestimated prevalence given the possibility that some students concealed their smoking status. A study conducted in Korea on the reliability of self-reported smoking behavior and found that many students hide their smoking behavior resulting in underestimated prevalence [23].

Our study indicates that male sex was positively associated with smoking behavior. The same findings were reported by other studies where male gender was significant risk factor for smoking [14–17]. Based on the present study, good knowledge showed a weak protective effect against being smoker while the effect of attitude was a strong. This agrees with a study on the effect of knowledge and attitude on smoking behavior in India where found similar findings and emphasized the importance of focusing on attitudes and belief rather than merely knowledge [13]. A good knowledge did not essentially translate into an appropriate behavior which is similar to other research' findings in the literature on effect of knowledge on practice [24].

This study found that presence of someone in the social environment such as family member or friends who smokes was risk factor of smoking behavior. This agrees with similar findings of two studies on determinants and risk factors of smoking behavior among university students in Turkey where having at least one immediate family member who smokes was risk factor for smoking [15, 16].

#06.2 Indonesia
Smoking behavior among university students in Germany and Indonesia: a comparative study

The present study found that receiving at least one kind of smoking promotions was significant risk factor for smoking. A similar findings by Chief Economic Advisor of the Department of Health of the Government of Great Britain which observed that limits on tobacco advertising tend to reduce tobacco usage beyond what would have happened in the absence of such a ban, and that advertising tends to encourage use of tobacco products[25].

CONCLUSION. There are several factors determining smoking behavior among university students including social factors and awareness level about potential health risks. Successful smoking prevention programs should consider the social environment's influence on the start and maintenance of smoking behavior, including the effect of parents, peers, and friends. Effective anti-smoking campaigns should intentionally target people's beliefs and attitudes and aim to persuade people and change their behavior, rather than simply delivering information. Anti-smoking policies should take into account the effect of tobacco advertisements and promotional activities.—

REFERENCES

1 World Health Organisation, W. Tobacco control. 2022 [cited 2022 16.12]; Available from: https://www.who.int/europe/news-room/fact-sheets/item/tobacco. **2** Spatial, temporal, and demographic patterns in prevalence of smoking tobacco use and attributable disease burden in 204 countries and territories, 1990-2019: a systematic analysis from the Global Burden of Disease Study 2019. Lancet, 2021. 397(10292): p. 2337-2360. **3** Kotz, D., M. Böckmann, and S. Kastaun, The Use of Tobacco, E-Cigarettes, and Methods to Quit Smoking in Germany. Dtsch Arztebl Int, 2018. 115(14): p. 235-242. **4** Heilert, D. and A. Kaul, Smoking Behaviour in Germany: Evidence from the SOEP. SSRN Electronic Journal, 2017. **5** Bafunno, D., et al., Tobacco control in Europe: A review of campaign strategies for teenagers and adults. Crit Rev Oncol Hematol, 2019. 138: p. 139-147. **6** Holipah, H., H.W. Sulistomo, and A. Maharani, Tobacco smoking and risk of all-cause mortality in Indonesia. PLoS One, 2020. 15(12): p. e0242558. **7** Sinha, D., Global Adult Tobacco Survey: Indonesia Report 2011. 2011. **8** (Indonesia)., M.o.H., Indonesia Health Profile 2014. 2015, Jakarta, Indonesia: Ministry of Health (Indonesia): Internet. **9** Nyman, A.L., T.M. Taylor, and L. Biener, Trends in cigar smoking and perceptions of health risks among Massachusetts adults. Tob Control, 2002. 11 Suppl 2(Suppl 2): p. ii25-8. **10** Hyland, A., et al., Individual-level predictors of cessation behaviours among participants in the International Tobacco Control (ITC) Four Country Survey. Tob Control, 2006. 15 Suppl 3(Suppl 3): p. iii83-94. **11** Raina, R., et al., Knowledge, attitude and behavioral determinants of tobacco use among 13-15 year old school children. J Int Soc Prev Community Dent, 2015. 5(4): p. 321-6. **12** Kimuyu, P., The Impact of Knowledge, Attitude and Social Norm Changes on Cigarette Smoking Behavior in the United States. München, GRIN Verlag, 2018: p. 10. **13** Nurmansyah, M.I., et al., Knowledge, attitude and practice of cigarette smoking among senior secondary school students in Depok, Indonesia. Int J Adolesc Med Health, 2019. 33(2). **14** Nasser, A.M.A. and X. Zhang, Knowledge and factors related to smoking among university students at Hodeidah University, Yemen. Tob Induc Dis, 2019. 17: p. 42. **15** Oncel, S., O. Gebizlioglu, and F. Aliev, Risk factors for smoking behavior among university students. Turkish Journal of Medical Sciences, 2011. 41. **16** Karadoğan, D., Ö. Önal, and Y. Kanbay, Prevalence and determinants of smoking status among university students: Artvin Çoruh University sample. PLoS One, 2018. 13(12): p. e0200671. **17** Al-Kubaisy, W., et al., Factors Associated with Smoking Behaviour among University Students in Syria. Procedia - Social and Behavioral Sciences, 2012. 38: p. 59-65. **18** Dania, M.G., O.B. Ozoh, and E.O. Bandele, Smoking habits, awareness of risks, and attitude towards tobacco control policies among medical students in Lagos, Nigeria. Ann Afr Med, 2015. 14(1): p. 1-7. **19** Husten, C.G.,

Smoking cessation in young adults. Am J Public Health, 2007. 97(8): p. 1354-6. **20** Society, A.C. Why People Start Smoking and Why It's Hard to Stop. 2022 [cited 2022 16.12]; Available from: https://www.cancer.org/healthy/stay-away-from-tobacco/why-people-start-using-tobacco.html. **21** CDC, C.f.D.C.a.P. Definition of smoking status. 2022 [cited 2022; Available from: https://www.cdc.gov/nchs/nhis/tobacco/tobacco_glossary.htm **22** Al-Naggar, R.A., et al., Prevalence and of smoking and associated factors among Malaysian University students. Asian Pac J Cancer Prev, 2011. 12(3): p. 619-24. **23** Hwang, J.H., et al., Underestimation of Self-Reported Smoking Prevalence in Korean Adolescents: Evidence from Gold Standard by Combined Method. Int J Environ Res Public Health, 2018. 15(4). **24** Pang, J., S.W. Chua, and L. Hsu, Current knowledge, attitude and behaviour of hand and food hygiene in a developed residential community of Singapore: a cross-sectional survey. BMC Public Health, 2015. 15: p. 577. **25** Institute of Medicine (US) Committee on Preventing Nicotine Addiction in Children and Youths, L.B., Bonnie RJ, editors, Growing up Tobacco Free: Preventing Nicotine Addiction in Children and Youths. TOBACCO ADVERTISING AND PROMOTION, ed. B.R. Lynch BS, editors. 1994, Washington (DC): National Academies Press (US).

AUTHORS

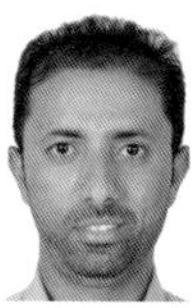

Hani Nasr
Research Associate Institute for Research in International Assistance (IRIA) | Akkon Hochschule für Humanwissenschaften | E-mail: Hani.Nasr@iria.akkon-hochschule,de

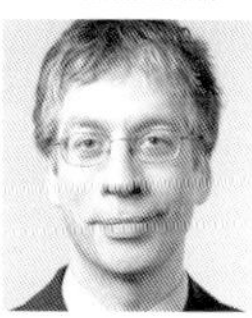

Prof. Dr. med. Dr. PH Timo Ulrichs
Head of Institute for Research in International Assistance (IRIA) | Akkon Hochschule für Humanwissenschaften | E-mail: timo.ulrichs@iria.akkon-hochschule.de

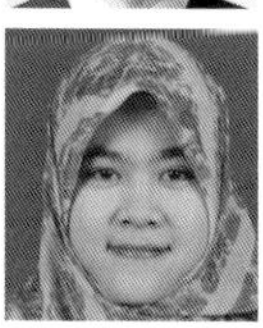

Nida Amalia
Faculty of Public Health | UMKT; Indonesia |
E-mail: na844@umkt.ac.id

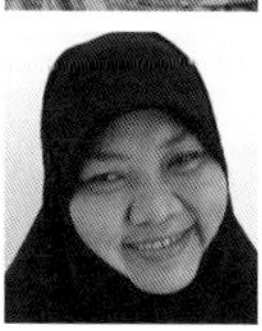

Sri Sunarti
Faculty of Public Health | UMKT; Indonesia |
E-mail: ss678@umkt.ac.id

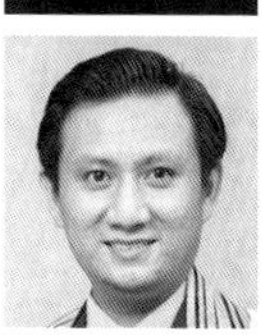

Kresna Febriyanto
Faculty of Public Health | UMKT; Indonesia |
E-mail: kresna.kesmas@umkt.ac.id

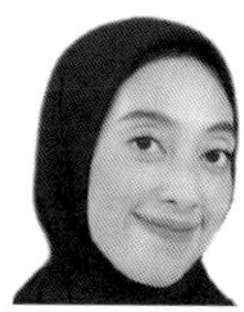

Erliga Nur Hikmah
Faculty of Public Health | UMKT; Indonesia |
E-mail: erliga05@umkt.ac.id

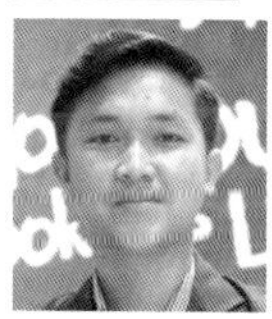

Gandi Puad Pratama
Faculty of Public Health | UMKT, Indonesia | E-mail: gandipuadpratama07@umkt.ac.id

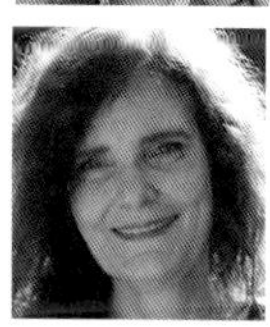

Gaby Feldmann, Dipl.-Geogr.
Co-Head Institute for Research in International Assistance (IRIA) | Akkon Hochschule für Humanwissenschaften
E-Mail: gaby.feldmann@iria.akkon-hochschule.de

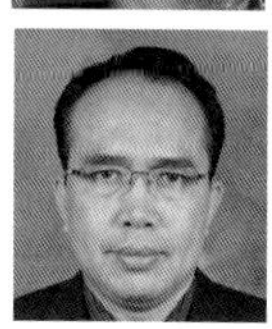

Ghozali
Faculty of Public Health | UMKT; Indonesia | E-mail: gm760@umkt.ac.id

Universitas Muhammadiyah Kalimantan Timur (UMKT)
Samarinda, Indonesia
E-mail: nidaamalia@umkt.ac.id

Akkon Hochschule für Humanwissenschaften/Institute for Research in International Assistance (IRIA), Berlin, Germany | E-mail: info@iria.akkon-hochschule.de

#06.3 Indonesia / South East Asia
Avian Influenza
Joana Kochendörfer

Avian influenza (derived from the Latin word "avis" for bird) is a viral disease that is considered the worst outbreak ever known in animals. A distinction is made between low-pathogenic (causing mild disease, LPAI) and highly pathogenic (causing severe disease, HPAI) viruses. The majority of poultry die once they become infected with the highly pathogenic virus. The virus usually spreads through infected feces, meaning that wild birds, especially waterfowl, already carry the virus, mostly in their gastrointestinal tract or respiratory system. However, since only LPAI viruses are present there, these birds usually do not get sick themselves, or only in a very mild form. However, since the viruses can survive for several weeks, protected by organic material (especially feces), they spread through the ingestion of feces by other birds (cf. Abrell n.d.).

The influenza A viruses are named after their structure and are divided into subtypes that differ in their surface proteins. There are 16 different H subtypes (hemagglutinin proteins) and nine different N subtypes (neuraminidase proteins). While all subtypes can occur in wild birds, subtypes H5 and H7 cause avian influenza, which primarily affects domestic poultry, and subtypes H1, H2, and H3 are the causative agents of human influenza (cf. Abrell n.d.).

Since the incubation period is longer than for "normal" human influenza (2–4 days), symptoms in humans may only occur after 14 days. Initially, the symptoms resemble those of the flu, with patients experiencing high fever, cough, sore throat, and difficulty breathing. In the further course of the disease, pneumonia, gastrointestinal problems, or elevated liver values often occur. In addition, a severe reduction in leukocytes weakens the immune system, the oxygen transport capacity of the blood is reduced by a significant reduction in erythrocytes, and spontaneous bleeding occurs repeatedly due to the strong reduction in platelets. As a result, many patients die from fatal lung or multi-organ failure.

Since the virus occurs mainly in Asia, the Foreign Office warns travelers against it. They are advised to stay away from poultry markets and to avoid any contact with dead birds. In addition, only well-cooked meat should be eaten, as the virus is no longer infectious at temperatures above 70°C (cf. Foreign Office 2022).

SITUATION IN SOUTHEAST ASIA. According to the WHO, over 2,300 cases of human avian influenza have been reported worldwide since 2003, with most cases occurring in Asia and Egypt. So far, about 850 people have been infected with A(H5N1), of whom more than half have died, with 450 deaths reported. In March 2013, the WHO first reported the emergence of a new avian influenza virus, A(H7N9), in China. Although this variant is considered LPAI for birds, more than 1,500 people in China have been infected with A(H7N9) since then, of whom at least 600 have died (as of 2021). It has also been found that individual cases have been imported from China to Hong Kong, Macao, Taiwan, Canada, and Malaysia. Infections occur in waves, usually in the winter months. Since the majority of human cases can be attributed to visits to poultry markets, these have been closed in China since 2017 (cf. RKI 2018).

With 168 deaths since 2003, Indonesia leads the list of A(H5N1) fatalities, followed by Egypt and Vietnam. China ranks fifth with 31 deaths (as of 2020) (cf. Radtke 2022). Although in June 2021 the first A(H10N3) infection in a human was detected in China, currently no new infections of any variant in humans are known in China, Vietnam, Thailand or Indonesia (as of February 2023). However, in China, a new infection of the A(H5N1) variant was detected in 200 birds. Additionally, there was another case of this variant in Japan (cf. WHO 2023).—

REFERENCES

1 Abrell, Barbara (o.J.): Fakten zur Vogelgrippe [online], https://www.mpg.de/vogelgrippe [22.04.2022] **2** Auswärtiges Amt (2022): Vogelgrippe- Aviare Influenza [online], https://www.auswaertiges-amt.de/blob/254348/7a71975bb8eb85b7c95551b7e9024859/vogelgrippe-data.pdf [22.04.2022] **3** Radtke Rainer (2022): Influenza H5N1-Todesfälle nach Ländern weltweit bis 2022 [online], https://de.statista.com/statistik/daten/studie/1100709/umfrage/influenza-h5n1-todesfaelle-nach-laendern-weltweit/ [22.04.2022] **4** RKI (2018): Das RKI zu humanen Erkrankungsfällen mit aviärer Infuenza A(H7N9) [online], https://www.rki.de/DE/Content/InfAZ/Z/ZoonotischeInfluenza/InfluenzaA_H7N9.html [22.04.2022] **5** WHO (2023): Avian Influenza Weekly Update Number 889, [online] https://www.who.int/docs/defaultsource/wpro---documents/emergency/surveillance/avian-influenza/ai_20230331.pdf?sfvrsn=5bc7c406_23 [04.04.2023]

AUTHOR

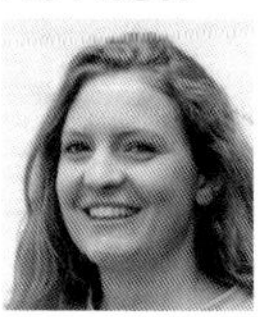

Joana Kochendörfer
Second year student International Emergency and Disaster Relief
Akkon Hochschule für Humanwissenschaften

#07 Iran
Investigating the role of self-efficacy and dysfunctional attitudes on psychological well-being in individuals with transgender
Zahra Taherian, Maryam Janfada, Arefeh Ranjbar, Iran

ABSTRACT. BACKGROUND. Transgenders often results in an insidious and permanent conflict within the person, a persistent feeling of discomfort with their assigned sex and of not fitting their biological and social role along with a constant desire to reassign to the gender and they are exposed to higher levels of discrimination, due to their rejection of the gender binary, which may be related to the development of psychopathologies.

AIMS. The present study aimed to investigate the role of self-efficacy and dysfunctional attitudes on psychological well-being of individuals with transgender.

METHOD. The method of present study was descriptive and correlational. The statistical population of the study included all individuals with sexual dissatisfaction in Mashhad in 2021. They were selected based on a convenience (voluntary) sampling method. For this purpose, the link of the online questionnaire was distributed in Telegram and WhatsApp cyberspace groups related to these individuals and 200 questionnaires were entered into the analysis. The instruments used in the study included Ryff Psychological Well-Being Scale (1989), the Scherer Self-Efficacy Scale (1891), and the Weissman and Beck (1978) Dysfunctional Attitudes Scale. For data analysis, Pearson correlation and simultaneous regression analysis were analyzed in SPSS-26 software.

RESULTS. The results of multiple regression showed that self-efficacy and dysfunctional attitudes could predict the psychological well-being of transgenders . The results of coefficient of explanation showed that self-efficacy and dysfunctional attitudes in transgenders could explain 46% of the changes in psychological well-being of the individuals. Regression coefficients also showed that self-efficacy had the greatest effect on predicting psychological well-being.

DISCUSSION. Thus, it can be stated that self-efficacy and dysfunctional attitudes have an effect on the psychological well-being of transgenders and these variables can be considered to prevent mental disorders and increase the efficiency and psychological well-being of these individuals.

KEYWORDS. Self-efficacy, Dysfunctional Attitudes, Psychological Well-being, Transgender

INTRODUCTION. The International Statistical Classification of Diseases, 10th revision (ICD-10) of the World Health

Organisation (WHO) uses the term transsexualism to describe the persistent manifestation of personal conflict between gender assigned at birth and felt gender. In the latest revision of this tool, the ICD-11, transsexualism was removed from the chapter on mental disorders and added to the chapter "Conditions Related to Sexual Health," and the use of the term "gender incongruence" was proposed. In the Diagnostic and Statistical Manual of Mental Disorders, Fifth Edition (DSM-5), however, transsexuality remains within categories of mental disorders with the term "gender dysphoria". Although the WHO "depathologizes" transsexuality, some transgender people may suffer discomfort or unease (dysphoria) because of this conflict. They may also experience symptoms resulting from minority stress and, as a result, they may develop associated psychopathology or psychiatric problems (Modrego Pardo et al., 2021).

Transsexuality often results in an insidious and permanent conflict within the person, a persistent feeling of discomfort with their assigned sex and of not fitting their biological and social role along with a constant desire to reassign to the gender with which they identify psychologically (Casado-Morente et al., 2021).

Transgender individuals, as a minority group, suffer from discrimination that negatively affects almost every life domain, severely impacting their social, medical, and psychological wellbeing. To this regard, religious fundamentalism (RF) has been described as one of the possible cultural features facilitating prejudice and negative attitudes toward transgender people, as well as internalized transphobia (Kanamori & Xu, 2020). Along those lines, the literature describes further difficulties regarding the social acceptance of gender diverse individuals; in fact, gender diverse individuals might experience the additional stigma of falling outside the societal binary norms, leading to challenges such as the use of pronouns and titles (Thorne et al., 2019). In addition, they are exposed to higher levels of discrimination, due to their rejection of the gender binary, which may be related to the development of psychopathologies (Monro, 2019). In particular (Romani et al., 2021), described that gender-diverse people generally experience greater levels of depression and anxiety compared to B ones, even though other studies do not report such differences (Rimes et al., 2019). The higher prevalence of psychopathologies such as depression and anxiety – seems to be driven by the lack of social support or, at the very least, by the lower visibility and comprehension of gender diverse identification (Thorne et al., 2019).

In recent years, transgender activism has led to greater recognition of transgender individuals (TSI) by the medical profession. Nevertheless, TSI faces discrimination and social stigma in everyday life. Furthermore, barriers to sex reassignment treatment and healthcare, in general, are described as an issue by many TSI (Pöge et al., 2020). These experiences as part of a gender or sexual minority can cause stress and consequently lead to a lower level of life satisfaction, impair mental health and increase the risk of developing psychiatric disorders (Kota et al., 2020).

Under such circumstances, it is necessary to pay attention to the psychological well-being of transgenders. Psychological wellbeing is a key indicator of general health. Psychological wellbeing is generally defined as a subjective experience of positive affections and life satisfaction. This construct has been also defined as positive psychological performance, good relations with others, and feeling realistic about self (McAneney et al., 2015). Studies have shown that psychological wellbeing is a multidimensional concept, which is created by the integration of emotion regulation, personality traits, identity, and life experiences. Individuals who have low psychological well-being feelings evaluate life events and situations undesired and experience negative emotions, such as anxiety, depression, and anger (Sharifian et al., 2020). It is useful to identify variables related to psychological wellbeing due to its positive aspects in Transgenders individuals.

Transgender individuals face significant challenges when deciding to cope with their personal, mental, behavioral, emotional, social, and educational problems and issues. Hence, self-efficacy is one of the critical cases that influence the psychological well-being of these individuals. Self-efficacy indicates the extent of a person's confidence in their abilities to perform a set of actions or a specific task. Self-efficacy also is the sense of competency, adequacy, and ability to cope with life. Self-efficacy beliefs include an important aspect of human motivation, behavior, and activities that can influence a person's life (Mizutani et al., 2012). Self-efficacy is a concept derived from an extensive theory called cognitive-social theory in which, personal achievement is influenced by behavior, environmental conditions, and inner characteristics, such as thoughts and beliefs (Eden et al., 2016). Individuals who have clear, defined, harmonic, and stable self-efficacy beliefs have higher psychological well-being. These individuals have reached an obvious perspective and are less influenced by daily events and relevant assessments of these incidents (Hosseini Dowlatabadi et al., 2014). On the other hand, low self-efficacy is correlated to increased mental pressure, weak responses to pain and suffering, and low motivation to pursue health-related programs; on contrary, high self-efficacy is correlated with lower mental pressure, fewer biological responses to mental pressures, higher adaptation power, interest in health programs, and higher responsibility (Delforooz et al.,

2021). Borg and Barlow (2018) showed that self-efficacy with personal management and control could increase psychological wellbeing.

Dysfunctional attitudes can also affect the psychological well-being level of Transgender individuals. Psychological wellbeing originates from cognitive and emotional evaluation of individuals in life, and what society people consider happiness, peace, prospect, and life satisfaction influence their psychological wellbeing (Delforooz et al., 2021). As a cognitive construct, dysfunctional attitudes play a vital role in psychological wellbeing; these attitudes and beliefs that are obtained from experience towards self and the world make an individual ready to interpret specific situations extremely negative and dysfunctional (Sharifian et al., 2020). Individuals who have pessimistic attitudes towards life issues always see themselves in unpleasant incidents and probably put themselves at risk of diseases (Wang et al., 2017). Dysfunctional attitudes are activated immediately after negative events of life and activate information processing patterns with negative orientation. These are considered, as a negative factor for individuals' wellbeing (Babayan, 2017). Researchers believe that dysfunctional attitudes severely decrease wellbeing by creating unnecessary emotional disorders (Yung, 2017). Sari (2022) indicated that dysfunctional attitudes indirectly led to worry, unhappiness, and depression. These beliefs increase negative self-judgments, loss of confidence, underestimation of abilities and achievements, sense of dissatisfaction, depression, and anxiety. Perez and Rohan (2021) in a study with gender control indicated that dysfunctional attitudes considerably predicted new depression intensity. Yung (2017) found a positive and significant relationship between dysfunctional attitudes and negative wellbeing indicators, such as depression and anxiety, and found a negative correlation between dysfunctional attitudes and positive wellbeing indicators, such as life satisfaction. Park et al. (2013) found a negative relationship between dysfunctional attitudes and quality of life. Tehranchi et al. (2018) indicated a positive association between dysfunctional attitudes and negative wellbeing indicators (depression), and a negative relationship between dysfunctional attitudes and positive wellbeing indicators (happiness, hope).

As mentioned about specific problems and conditions in the life of transgender individuals, it is important to investigate the factors affecting their psychological wellbeing to prevent mental disorders and enhance the psychological wellbeing and efficiency of these individuals. Therefore, the extant study aimed to examine the impact of self-efficacy and dysfunctional attitudes on the psychological wellbeing of transgenders.

METHOD. The extant study was descriptive with correlational type. The statistical population of the study comprised all individuals with sexual dissatisfaction living in Mashhad (2021). The subjects were chosen using a convenience sampling method. For this purpose, the online questionnaire's link designed in the Avval Form website was sent in virtual groups of studied individuals; of them, 215 members filled out the questionnaires. After incomplete questionnaires were removed, data of 200 subjects were analyzed. Inclusion criteria were as follows: being Transgender, voluntarily participating in the study and complete answers given to questions. Lack of transgenderism and appropriate response were exclusion criteria. In this research, questionnaires were designed through the online method in the Avval Form website then sent to virtual networks, Telegram, and WhatsApp groups of participants to fill the questionnaires out.

RESEARCH INSTRUMENTS.

Ryff Scales of Psychological Well-Being (PWB)

This scale was designed by Ryff to assess psychological wellbeing components, and consisted of 84 items and PWB areas: self-acceptance, positive relations with others, autonomy, environmental mastery, purpose in life, and personal growth. This questionnaire is scored based on the Likert scale from strongly disagree (1) to strongly agree (2). Of all items, 44 items were directly rated, while 40 items were scored indirectly. Ryff (1989) in a study on adolescents and adult people obtained reliability between 0.86 and 0.93 for considered factors, which implied suitable validity and reliability of the test. Bayani et al. (2008) examined this scale on a 145-member sample of students, and reliability results through retest equaled 0.82, 0.71, 0.77, 0.78, 0.77, 0.70, and 0.78 for the total score, self-acceptance, positive relations with others, autonomy, environmental mastery, purpose in life, and personal growth, respectively. Life satisfaction, Oxford happiness, and Rosenberg's Self-Esteem scales were used to examine validity; the correlation between the PWB scale and the mentioned questionnaire equaled 0.47, 0.58, and 0.46, respectively.

Shearer's Self-Efficacy Scale

This questionnaire was constructed by Sherer et al. (1981) and included 23 items of which, 17 items examine general self-efficacy and 6 items test self-efficacy experiences in social situations. The 17-item scale was used in the extant study. Self-efficacy scale measures personal beliefs, and a person's ability to overcome different situations. This questionnaire has been designed based on the five-point Likert scale (from strongly disagree (1) to strongly agree (5)). The higher the score, the higher the sense of self-efficacy of a person will be; therefore, maximum and minimum scores of scale equal 85 and 17, respectively. Sherer et al. (1982) obtained Cronbach's alpha coefficient of 0.86 for this scale. Asgharnejad and colleagues (2006) validated this scale. The translated version of this scale was filled out by 344 students. Exploratory and confirmatory factor analyses were used to examine validity. The results of exploratory factor analysis indicated three factors and the results of confirmatory factor analysis were confirmed. Moreover, Cronbach's alpha was used to test the reliability of the scale and equaled 0.83. The extant study obtained Cronbach's alpha of 0.85 for this scale

Dysfunctional Attitude Scale (DAS-26)

This scale was designed by Weissman and Beak (1978). DAS consists of 26 items that are scored at a seven-point Likert scale from strongly disagree (1) to strongly agree (7). This scale includes four subscales: perfectionism, need for approval, need for satisfying others, and vulnerability. Various studies have reported mean scores between 119 and 128 for healthy people; the higher the score, the higher the vulnerability. Weissman et al. (1978) carried out a primary study on the development and validation of DAS. The results showed that DAS was constructed to measure the extensive negative attitude of a depressed person towards self, the world, and the future. DAS follows a cognitive disorder structure. This scale was derived from a 40-item version of Form A in 2012 to be used in the clinical population and determine its psychometric quality. The Iranian version of this scale is one the most famous instruments in cognitive studies, and comprises 26 items measuring four factors: perfectionism, need for approval, need for satisfying others, and vulnerability. The validity and reliability of this test had Cronbach's alpha of 0.85 with construct validity of 0.47 in normal and clinical populations.

The data collected from descriptive and inferential indicators (Pearson correlation coefficient and simultaneous regression) were analyzed through SPSS-26 software. It is worth noting that the general aim of the study was explained, and participants were ensured about information confidentiality in terms of ethical considerations.

RESULTS. In this research, 200 Transgender individuals participated. The age average of participants equaled 22.44 and a standard deviation of 6.80. Among participants, 25 members (12.5%) were female and 168 members (84%) were male, and 7 members (3.5%) were non-binary; 26 participants (23%) had an associate degree, 87 members (43.5%) had diploma, 65 members (32.5%) had BA degree, and 2 members (1%) had MA degree. Table 1 reports the mean value, standard de-

Variable	Mean	SD	1	2	3	4	5	6	7
1. self-efficacy	69.64	8.77	1						
2. perfectionism	30.29	10.53	-0.55**	1					
3. need for approval	12.35	5.17	-0.49**	0.64**					
4. need for satisfying others	17.97	5.82	-0.42**	0.80**	0.57**	1			
5. vulnerability	17.91	4.91	0.26**	0.06	-0.00	0.15*			
6. dysfunctional attitudes	75.01	20.17	-0.48**	0.91**	0.78**	0.85**	0.27**	1	
7. psychological wellbeing	217.86	22.40	0.63**	-0.38**	-0.28**	-0.30**	0.36**	-0.29**	1

Table 1. Mean and standard deviation of research variables.

viation, and correlation coefficient between research variables.

The results of the correlation coefficient indicated a negative and positive significant correlation between psychological wellbeing and dysfunctional attitudes (-0.29) and self-efficacy (0.63), respectively. Furthermore, the results showed a negative significant correlation (-0.48) between dysfunctional attitudes and self-efficacy.

Multiple regression techniques were used to examine the role of self-efficacy and dysfunctional attitudes in predicting the psychological wellbeing of transgender individuals. Normality (using skewness and kurtosis), collinearity of variables (variance inflation factor and tolerance index), and errors independence (Durbin-Watson test) assumptions were examined before model testing. Table 2 presents the results of presumptions.

Variable	Skewness	Kurtosis	Tolerance index	Tolerance index
Self-efficacy	1.88	1.85	0.58	1.72
Perfectionism	1.17	0.28	0.28	2.61
Need for approval	0.29	0.70	0.55	1.82
Need for satisfying others	2.11	1.91	0.43	2.91
Vulnerability-performance evaluation	1.81	1.32	0.84	1.18

Table 2. Results of skewness and kurtosis, tolerance index, and variance inflation factor (VIF).

It is better to use skewness and kurtosis for normality reports due to the large sample size. Therefore, skewness and kurtosis were used for normality presumption. Skewness and kurtosis values were measured by calculating Z (Skewness and kurtosis index divided by error). The z values less than 2.5 indicate the normal distribution of variables. According to the results of skewness and kurtosis, all values were lower than 2.5; hence, the variables were normal. The tolerance index of all variables equaled 0.9, and the inflation index was less than ten (VIF<10); moreover, the D-W value equaled 1.83, which was less than 4. Hence, presumptions were not violated. Therefore, the measured indicators indicated that test conditions were observed. Results of multiple regression implementations have been reported in Table 3.

According to the results of implemented multiple regression, self-efficacy and dysfunctional variables could predict the psychological wellbeing of Transgenders ($F=32.72$, $p<0.05$). Moreover, the results showed that coefficient of determination (R2) equaled 0.46 implying that self-efficacy and dysfunctional attitudes of transgenders could predict 46% of variations in their psychological wellbeing. Results of multiple regression analysis examined mixed effects of predictors on criterion variables. Therefore, regression coefficient results are reported to find which variable can predict psychological wellbeing.

As it is seen, standardized coefficients of regression indicated that self-efficacy could predict psychological wellbeing positively and significantly while performance evaluation could negatively and significantly predict psychological wellbeing in transgenders. The results obtained from standardized coefficients of regression indicated that self-efficacy had the highest effect (ß=0.52) on psychological wellbeing.

Source of variations	Sum of squares	df	Mean squares	R^2	F	Sig.
Self-efficacy	45713.34	5	9142.66	0.46	32.72	0.000
Perfectionism	51198.01	194	279.37			
Need for approval	99911.35	199				

Table 3. Results of regression implementation to predict psychological wellbeing symptoms based on self-efficacy and dysfunctional attitudes.

#07 Iran
Investigating the role of self-efficacy and dysfunctional attitudes on psychological well-being in individuals with transgender

Predictor variable	Regression coefficients (ß)	SD error	Standardized coefficients of regression (ß	t	Sig.
Self-efficacy	1.33	0.17	0.52	7.55	0.000
Perfectionism	-0.19	0.21	-0.09	-0.90	0.368
Need for approval	0.39	0.31	0.09	1.26	0.209
Need for satisfying others	-0.36	0.34	-0.09	-1.03	0.301
Vulnerability-performance evaluation	-1.10	0.26	-0.24	-4.22	0.000

Table 4. Standardized coefficients of regression.

DISCUSSION AND CONCLUSION. The extant study aimed to examine the impact of self-efficacy on the psychological well-being of transgenders. The results of data indicated that these variables could predict psychological wellbeing in transgenders, and self-efficacy and dysfunctional attitudes could explain 46% of changes in psychological well-being. Results of regression coefficients showed that self-efficacy and dysfunctional attitude of performance evaluation could predict psychological well-being of transgenders; self-efficacy had the highest role in the prediction of psychological wellbeing.

The first result showed the positive impact of self-efficacy on psychological wellbeing, which was matched with findings obtained by Matteucci and Soncini (2021), Kennis et al. (2021), Li and Feng (2018), Borg and Barlow (2018), Eeri et al. (2018), Kolahi et al. (2019), and Sevari (2020). The mentioned studies indicated that's self-efficacy could predict psychological wellbeing. Hashemi and Ahmadi (2015) carried out a study and showed that self-efficacy and Masculinity-Feminity gender roles could predict psychological hardiness. This result can be explained based on Bandura's theory in which, self-efficacy can determine how a person copes with life tasks and respective stresses. In other words, individuals' beliefs about their capabilities and eligibilities to apply a set of actions to achieve a desired level of performance encourage them to encounter life challenges and acquire valuable experiences (Bandura, 1997). Self-efficacy affects how to cope with problems, emotional health, decision-making, and dealing with stress (Seggelen & Van Dam, 2016). Self-efficacy is a cognitive mediator that influences thoughts and feelings. Transgenders experience many problems; therefore, a high sense of self-efficacy helps them to manage negative events and stressful situations and protect themselves when experiencing such incidents. Such high-rate self-efficacy leads to higher psychological well-being among transgender individuals. Moreover, it can be explained that self-efficacy is a personal factor that its high level allows the person to enjoy the performance, existing conditions, and their activities paying attention to their good inner senses towards them.

In terms of the impact of dysfunctional attitudes on psychological wellbeing, research findings are consistent with results obtained by Sari (2022), Perez and Rohan (2021), Park et al. (2013), Tehranchi et al. (2018), Zorrahim and Beyrami (2015). Perez and Rohan (2021) conducted a study with gender control and showed that dysfunctional attitudes could considerably predict the next depression rate, while none of the cognitive vulnerabilities to negative events of life were significant for depression prediction. In this case, Brouwer et al. (2019) indicated that dysfunctional attitudes make a person prone to psychological disorders. Dysfunctional beliefs in life may be created by early experiences in the field of risks and pains that come to the person and finally lead to chronic and unpleasant behavioral patterns. In other words, dysfunctional attitudes reflect perceptions of self, others, and life events (Zawadzki et al., 2020).

It can be explained that dysfunctional attitudes are considered as a vulnerability factor under stressful environmental conditions and unpleasant events or negative experiences over life leads to the creation of dysfunctional assumptions and attitudes in person (Beck, 2011). Vulnerable individuals evaluate any kind of new information and experiences based on negative beliefs and select the information that strengthens and confirms these beliefs (Beck, 2011). In this case, Rabiei et al. (2009) concluded that performance evaluation and social proof could explain 16% of the variance in mental health. It can be explained about the impact of performance evaluation vulnerability on the psychological wellbeing of transgenders that individuals with positive attitudes, hopeful, and free of intellectual errors have a creative and flexible view towards issues, and plan to solve these problems. They do not hesitate to ask others for help if required and have complete resources to cope with problems (Chen et al., 2019). The mentioned factors help a person to have higher mental health and psychological wellbeing and lower dysfunctional attitudes. It is concluded that a person's perception of the environment influences the behaviors, affections, and emotions of the individual. On the other hand, positive attitudes towards events and situations lead to positive emotions, which in turn bring psychological wellbeing.

#07 Iran
Investigating the role of self-efficacy and dysfunctional attitudes on psychological well-being in individuals with transgender

All studies face some constraints that reduce generalization. Because this study was conducted on Transgender society, findings cannot be generalized to other individuals of the society. Moreover, research findings were limited to data obtained from the self-report scale that were gathered through the online method. The absence of some instruments, such as an interview for data collection can be mentioned in the assessment of these variables. Because results indicated the important role of self-efficacy in predicting the psychological wellbeing of transgenders, it is recommended to consider the self-efficacy of these individuals in consultation and treatment cases. It is also suggested for further studies to examine and compare the increased self-efficacy and role of dysfunctional attitudes in transgenders before and after surgery.

FUNDING. This study was funded by X (grant number X).

CONFLICT OF INTEREST. The authors declare that they have no conflict of interest.

ETHICAL APPROVAL. All procedures performed in studies involving human participants were in accordance with the ethical standards of the institutional and/or national research committee and with the 1964 Helsinki declaration and its later amendments or comparable ethical standards.

INFORMED CONSENT. Informed consent was obtained from all individual participants included in the study.—

REFERENCES

Babayan, S. (2017). Study of the Relationship between Domain-Specific Hope and Dysfunctional Attitudes in Students of Islamic Azad University of Gorgan – Iran. Mediterranean Journal of Social Sciences, 6(1), 593-597. • Bandura, A. (1997). Self-efficacy: The Exercise of Control. New York, NY: Freeman. • Beck J. S. (2011). Cognitive behavior therapy: Basics and beyond. Guilford Press. • Borg, K., Barlow, J. (2018). The behaviors and perceptions of pediatricians in Malta relating to child protection work: National and international implications of a mixed-methods study. Child Abuse Review, 27(6), 446–467. • Brouwer, M. E., Williams, A. D., Forand, N. R., DeRubeis, R. J., & Bockting, C. L. H. (2019). Dysfunctional attitudes or extreme response style as predictors of depressive relapse and recurrence after mobile cognitive therapy for recurrent depression. Journal of Affective Disorders, 243, 48–54. • Casado-Morente, J. C., Mora Rivas, E., O'Connor Reina, C., Angulo Serrano, S., Díaz-Fresno, E., Sandoval-Menéndez, I., &Núñez-Batalla, F. (2021). Development and Validation of the Spanish Abbreviated Version of the Transsexual Voice Questionnaire for Male-to-Female Transsexuals. Acta Otorrinolaringologica, 72(1), 21–26. • Chen, A. M. H., Cailor, S., Franz, T., Fox, N., Thornton, P., & Norfolk, M. L. (2019). Development and validation of the self-care counseling rubric (SCCR) to assess student self-care counseling skills. Currents in Pharmacy Teaching and Learning, 11(8):774–781. • Delforooz, S., Ebrahimi, M., Mirhashemi, M., & Ghodsi, P. (2021). Develop a model of adolescent psychological well-being based on basic needs, parent-child relationship, and responsibility mediated by self-efficacy. Pajouhan Scientific Journal, 20(2), 63–70. | Eden, G. F., Olulade, O. A., Evans, T. M., Krafnick, A. J., & Alkire, D. R. (2016). Developmental dyslexia. In: Small GHL, editor. Neurobiology of language. San Diego: Academic Press, 815, 18–260. • Eeri, Y., Fakhri, M. K., & Hassanzadeh, R. (2018). Modeling structural relation between happiness and psychological wellbeing with the mediation of self-efficacy among students of Farhangian University. International Clinical Neuroscience Journal, 5(3), 273–281. • Hashemi, S., & Ahmadi, O. (2015).

Role of general self-efficacy and masculinity-feminity gender roles in psychological hardiness. Journal of Modern Psychological Researches, 10(37), 72–87. • Hosseini Dowlatabadi, F., Sadeghi, A., Saadat, S., & Khodayari, H. (2014). Relationship between self-efficacy and self-actualization with coping strategies among students. Research in Medical Education, 6(1), 10–18. • Kanamori, Y., & Xu, Y. J. (2020). Factors associated with transphobia: A structural equation modeling approach. Journal of Homosexuality, 15, 1–25. • Kennis, M., Duecker, F., T'Sjoen, G., Sack, A. T., & Dewitte, M. (2021). Sexual Self-Concept Discrepancies Mediate the Relation between Gender Dysphoria Sexual Esteem and Sexual Attitudes in Binary Transgender Individuals. The Journal of Sex Research, 1–13. doi: 10.1080/00224499.2021.1951643 • Kolahi, P., Aghel Masjedi, M., Mirghafari, S B., Rahmani, S., & Mohamadpour, S. (2019). The role of identity and self-efficacy styles in predicting psychological well-being. Islam and Health Journal, 4(2), 25–33. • Kota, K. K., Salazar, L. F., Culbreth, R. E., Crosby, R. A., & Jones, J. (2020). Psychosocial mediators of perceived stigma and suicidal ideation among transgender women. BMC Public Health, 29(1), 125. https://doi.org/10.1186/s12889-020-8177-z • Li, T., & Feng, F. (2018). Goal content, well-being, and psychological needs satisfaction in Chinese adolescents. Social Behavior and Personality: An International Journal, 46, 541-550. • Matteucci, M. C., & Soncini, A. (2021). Self-efficacy and psychological well-being in a sample of Italian university students with and without Specific Learning Disorder. Research in Developmental Disabilities, 110, 103–858. • McAneney, H., Tully, M. A., Hunter, R. F., Kouvonen, A., Veal, P., Stevenson, M., et al. (2015). Individual factors and perceived community characteristics about mental health and mental well-being. BMC Public Health, 15(1), 1237. • Mizutani, S., Ekuni, D., Furuta, M., Tomofuji, T., Irie, K., Azuma, T., & Morita, M. (2012). Effects of self-efficacy on oral health behaviors and gingival health in university students aged 18 or 19 years old. Journal of Clinical Periodontology, 39, 844–849. • Modrego Pardo, I., Gómez Balaguer, M., Hurtado Murillo, F., Cuñat Navarro, E., Solá Izquierdo, E., & Morillas Ariño, C. (2021). Self-injurious and suicidal behaviour in a transsexual adolescent and young adult population, treated at a specialised gender identity unit in Spain. Endocrinología, Diabetes y Nutrición, 68(5), 338–345. • Monro, S. (2019). Non-binary and genderqueer: An overview of the field. International Journal of Transgender, 20, 126–131. • Park, S. G., Bennett, M. E., Couture, S. M., & Blanchard, J. J. (2013). Internalized stigma in schizophrenia: Relations with dysfunctional attitudes, symptoms, and quality of life. Psychiatry Research, 205, 43–47. • Perez, J., & Rohan, K. J. (2021). Cognitive predictors of depressive symptoms. Cognitive reactivity, mood reactivity, and dysfunctional attitudes. Cognitive Therapy and Research, 45(1), 123–135. • Pöge, K., Dennert, G., Koppe, U., Güldenring, A., Matthigack, E. B., & Romme, A. (2020). The health of lesbian, gay, bisexual, transgender and intersex people.Journal of Health Monitoring, 5(S1), 2–27. https://doi.org/10.25646/6449 • Rabiei, M., Molavi, H., Kalantari, M., Azimi, H. (2009). The relationship between dysfunctional attitudes, coping strategies and mental health. New Educational Approaches, 4(2), 27–38. • Rimes, K. A., Goodship, N., Ussher, G., Baker, D., & West, E. (2019). Non-binary and binary transgender youth: Comparison of mental health, self-harm, suicidality, substance use, and victimization experiences. International Journal of Transgender, 20, 230–240. • Romani, A., Mazzoli, F., Ristori, J., Cocchetti, C., Cassioli, E., Castellini, G., & Fisher, A. D. (2021). Psychological Wellbeing and Perceived Social Acceptance in Gender Diverse Individuals. The Journal of Sexual Medicine, 18(11), 1933–1944. • Sari, E. A. H. I. (2022). Depression, Anxiety, and Stress in University Students: Effects of Dysfunctional Attitudes, Self-Esteem, and Age. Editorial Board, 12(1), 109. • Seggelen – Damen, I. V., & Van Dam, K. (2016). Self-Reflection as a Mediator between Self-Efficacy and Well-Being. Journal of Managerial Psychology, 31(1), 18–33. • Sevari, K. (2020). The mediating role of academic, social, and emotional self-efficacy in the relationship between cognitive flexibility and psychological well-being. Journal of Rooyesh, 9(5), 39–50. • Sharifian, M., Jandaghi, F., Nazarchoob Masjedi, M., Azizi, S. (2020). Mediating role of spiritual health in the relationship of irrational beliefs and dysfunctional attitudes with psychological well-being in a patient with multiple sclerosis by Structural equation modeling approach. Islamic Life Style Centered on Health, 4(2), 28–37. • Tehranchi, A., NeshatDoost, H.T., Amiri, S., Power, M.J. (2018). The Role of Character Strengths in Depression: A Structural Equation Model. Frontiers in Psychology, 9, 16-19. • Thorne, N., Witcomb, G. L., Nieder, T., Nixon, E., Yip, A., & Arcelus, J. (2019). A comparison of mental health symptomatology and levels of social support in young treatment seeking transgender individuals who identify as binary and non-binary. International Journal of Transgender, 20, 241–250. • Wang, C., Zhang, K., & Zhang, M. (2017). Dysfunctional attitudes learned helplessness, and coping styles among men with substance use disorders. Social Behavior and Personality: An International Journal, 45(2), 269–80. • Zawadzki, S. J., Bouman, T., Steg, L., Bojarskich, V., & Druen, P. B. (2020). Translating climate beliefs into action in a changing political landscape. Climatic Change, 161, 21–42. • Zorrahim, R., & Beyrami, M. (2016). Relationship between dysfunctional attitudes with the components of psychological well-being in students of the Islamic Azad University of Tabriz. Community Health Journal, 9(3), 9–17.

#07 Iran
Investigating the role of self-efficacy and dysfunctional attitudes on psychological well-being in individuals with transgender

AUTHORS

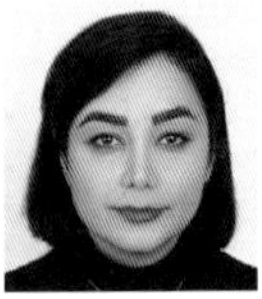

Zahra Taherian
Pronouns – she/her/hers
Master of counseling | Psychologist at Student Counseling and Social Work Center Ferdowsi University of Mashhad Manager of Senobar psychology clinic
Master of Counseling Family, Department of Psychology, Faculty of Education Science and Psychology, University of Ferdowsi, Mashhad, Iran, ifa fellow 2022
E-mail: mahla.taherian@gmail.com, ORCID: 0000-0002-3312-3408

Maryam Janfada
Master of General Psychology, Department of Psychology, Faculty of Education Science and Psychology, University of Ferdowsi, Mashhad, Iran, E-mail: ma.janfadah12@gmail.com, ORCID: 0000-0001-5040-2153

Arefeh Ranjbar
PhD student Educational Psychology, Department of Psychology, Faculty of Education Science and Psychology, University of Ferdowsi, Mashhad, Iran, E-mail: Arefeh.ranjbar@mail.um.ac.ir, ORCID: 0000-0003-3113-6325

#08 Philippines
Analyzing Gender Aspects of Teenage Pregnancy in the Philippines
Amelyn L. Laro, RSW, MASW

INTRODUCTION. The purpose of writing this research paper encompasses the following reasons: First, I will explain how teen pregnancy has become a major issue in the Philippines. Second, the researcher aims to fully understand how various texts discuss the causes and impact of teenage pregnancy. Third, as a social worker and gender advocate would like to analyze the intersectionality of how sociocultural components, health and psychological ramifications, educational systems, and technological advancements affect young teenage mothers, based on my experiences dealing with gender-sensitive cases. Finally, I will outline the implications of future directions on how Filipinos be more gender-sensitive in addressing teenage pregnancy in the Philippines.

METHODOLOGY. The qualitative method was used in this study. First is the literature review, which involves researching, reading, analyzing, evaluating, and summarizing scholarly literature (Paul and Criado, 2020. The articles and literature reviewed came from peer-reviewed journals, policy reports from international organizations, and published research. There are 30 literature reviews under the topic "teenage pregnancy" utilized in this study because of their relevance and suitability to the discussions. The information gathered was analyzed and synthesized. Specifically, this study utilized a semi-systematic or narrative review, which is more appropriate for topics that have been conceptualized differently and studied by various groups of researchers within diverse disciplines (Snyder, 2019). In addition, the use of a case study to analyze how such concepts are applied in the actual case encountered by the author.

RESULTS AND DISCUSSIONS.
Teenage pregnancy in the Philippines. The problem of teenage pregnancy in the Philippines is a phenomenon, and this is supported by several studies explaining how such a problem arises over a long period. According to the United Nations Population Fund (UNFPA), 16 million teenage girls between the ages of 15 and 19 and 2 million girls under the age of 15 become pregnant or give birth each year in the Philippines. This is aggravated by the problem of teenage pregnancy deaths, which is on the rise, according to the National Statistics Office (NSO) in Manila. Records indicated that the number increased to 10% in 2010 from 5% in 2000. (NSO, 2017). These girls' development is impacted because they are still developing when they give birth. Based on the study by Pogoy et al. (2014), teenage moms frequently experience developmental risk

factors, including cervical problems and stunted growth, which have a health-related impact. Other research has determined that teen motherhood invites social isolation, stigma, and prejudice in society (Cherry & Dillon, 2014; Smit-Battle, 2013). As a result, less than 2% of these girls graduate from college by the age of 30, which has an impact on their schooling as well (Natividad, 2014). J. N. Odhiambo (2018) Due to inadequate prenatal care, socioeconomic obstacles, and excessive weight gain during pregnancy, the prevalence of death in teenage pregnancies and poor birth outcomes is rising every year (Xi-Kuan, Shi Wu, Flemming Demissie, & Rhoads, 2007). Alvarez, M. O. C., Salvador, J. T., Sauce, B. R. J., and Rosario, A. B. (2016).
The risk of maternal mortality and delivery increases with teen pregnancy, including severe newborn problems, labor obstruction, systemic infections, stillbirth, and early birth. Teenage pregnancy also places young people at a greater disadvantage, including fewer job opportunities, lower school attainment, and negative health effects. As a result, they are more likely than other individuals to drop out of school. Cuisia-Cruz, E. S. S., Tabei, K., Smith, C., and Seposo, X. (2021). Teenage pregnancies have a variety of consequences, including a negative impact on the physical, emotional, social, and spiritual health of young people. The problem is linked to a variety of subsequent negative health and psychological effects. Based on the study of Marshall and Jones (2012), adolescent pregnancy is dangerous and lethal, with serious long-term effects that range from wider psychosocial concerns to health issues for the young mother and the child. Teenage mothers and their unborn children face medical dangers. A study by the World Health Organization (2012) revealed that women under the age of 20 are five times more likely than women over the age of 20 to die during pregnancy or childbirth. Pregnancy and childbirth increase the risk of morbidity and mortality in both children and mothers in this age group (NSO, 2009; WHO). This resulted in the deaths of more young women who gave birth in the country.
Since the phenomenon has become more common in recent years, some other causes identified for the high rise of this number identified three major themes: individual reasons (curiosity and inadequate sex knowledge, uncontrolled emotions, and retaliation), socio-cultural factors (peer influence, lack of parental guidance, culture, and transactional sex), and psychological repercussions (emotional reactions, fear, and low self-esteem). Morgan, A., Habito, C. M., and Vaughan (2021). Furthermore, low levels of education, dysfunctional families, and the underuse of medical resources contribute to this, according to Acharya, Bhattarai, Poobalan, and Chapman (2014). Some of the literature that

has been reviewed focuses on some of these important variables, which the author has classified as micro, mezzo, and macro causes: Micro-factors cover peer pressure and a lack of parental guidance, while mezzo-factors involve the use of technology and a lack of comprehensive sexuality education in schools, and macro-factors cover the cultural system, poverty, and the inefficiency of the government sector to address the problem.

Peer Pressures. One of the studies explains that teenage females were more likely to participate in early sexual conduct than their classmates, who did not hang out with such girls. Peers tend to have more impact than parents. However, a parent's presence and direction are crucial for a teen's development and social life. The realities in the Philippine context are that many parents are not communicating with their children about topics like sexuality and pregnancy, as these are considered taboo in some families with a conservative upbringing. Other factors that contribute to teen pregnancy include their families' willingness to engage in sexual activity with their boyfriends, as well as peer pressure or pressure from friends. Libo-on, J., O., F. Manzo, and I. Manzo (2021).

Lack of parental guidance. The study by Deptula, Henry, and Schoeny (2010) showed that low rates of teenage initiation of unprotected sex, pregnancy, and intercourse have been linked to high parental guidance. On the other hand, a strict upbringing can influence the desire to rebel, leave the house, and engage in sexual activities. A separate study confirmed that a combination of poor parental oversight and other factors contributed to this problem. J., O., F. Manzo, and I. Manzo (2021).

Lack of comprehensive sex education and misuse of social media platforms. A lack of education (Eloundou-Enyegue, 2004), Moreover, teenage pregnancies can occasionally come from adolescents who are lured by what they see in the media but lack knowledge about sex. According to Pogoy et al. (2014), having sex knowledge is crucial. Comparing adolescents who got thorough sex education to those who did not, the likelihood of teen pregnancy was much lower for the former group (Lindberg & Maddow-Zimet, 2012). O'Donnell, Myint-U, Duran, and Stueve (2010) noted that where girls' intervention programs were implemented, fewer reports of sexual risk behaviors were made. There are several explanations; for instance, Salvador, Sauce, Alvarez, and Rosario's (2016) study hypothesized that teen pregnancy is made more common by technology and that a lack of adolescent sexual and reproductive health education may be a factor in teenage pregnancy. Filipinos inhabit a society that is shaped by constantly evolving social trends. There are many different media outlets today. Everyone readily adopts what is typically the case and what is seen. Teenagers' activities, reactions to peer pressure, and behaviors are influenced by the usage of cell phones and ready access to multimedia. Television, radio, and even Internet-based information are key forms of communication and interaction among Filipino youths. They first communicated with each other over text messaging. Meeting up with them soon became routine, and eventually, they established intimate physical contact. This situation is typical of the city's overpopulated, low-wage workers. Morgan, A., Habito, C. M., and Vaughan (2021) explain that another important reason for the rise in teenage pregnancies is thought to be modern technology. Occasionally, teenagers get hooked on different social networking sites such as Facebook, online dating, Instagram, etc., utilizing their cell phones, notebooks, and tablets. Unplanned pregnancies frequently result from young people's curiosity and easy access to new technology, combined with their lack of information about family planning and contraception. In a country where most of its young people are using social media platforms like Instagram, Facebook, and TikTok increased the possibility of getting an online date and early sexual engagement will lead young women to be more prone to participate in unprotected sexual activities.

Cultural system in the country. According to Javier et al. (2010), culture has also contributed to the breakdown of mother-daughter communication and relationships. The same researchers also found that teenagers felt uncomfortable talking to their parents about sex issues because they worried that they might already be having sex (Javier et al., 2010). J. N. Poor mother-daughter communication is a known risk factor for early sex and probable conception, according to studies (Aruda, 2010; Dean, 2013). Adolescent girls may be influenced by dysfunctional parent-child interactions to seek caring relationships from their boyfriends. Pressure from such relationships eventually results in promiscuity and pregnancy (Javier, 2010). As Panday et al. (2014) indicated, it is evident from the literature that family structure traits are understood and responsible for teenage sexual activity, including pregnancy. J. N. Odhiambo (2018)

Impact of poverty and poor government interventions. Statistics confirm that teen pregnancy rates climb proportionately as one's socioeconomic standing declines (Pogoy et al., 2014). Moreover, data demonstrates that teens from poor families have a teenage pregnancy rate that is five times greater than the national norm (Berliner, 2013). The same study maintains that teen pregnancies are particularly common in deprived areas. The setting in which a teen lives and develops frequently has a big impact on their conduct. J. N. Odhiambo (2018) Teenage pregnancy is disproportionately common in low-income families for unknown reasons; as a result, young girls are often forced to engage in sex in exchange for money. Pogoy et al. (2014) confirmed the link between early sex and teenage pregnancy and familial and financial difficulties. Another researcher has concurred with the idea that adolescents' low socioeconomic situation correlates to adolescent pregnancy (Taffa & Obare, 2017).

Gender issues arise from teenage pregnancies. Numerous studies have identified a variety of factors that contribute to the causes and reasons why young female adolescents in the Philippines engage in sexual activity at an early age and how this leads to teenage pregnancy. As a school social worker, I see such phenomena not only as the result of the micro (peer pressures and a lack of parental guidance) and mezzo (poor use of technology and a lack of comprehensive sexuality education in schools) and macro (conservative cultural system, poor conditions, and government interventions to the problem), but it is also a classic example of a gender issue for young women. I will cite a concrete example from a case study that I encountered in my practice as a social worker.

The case of "Diva". She was a college student from the province who decided to study in Davao City. Her family's upbringing is deeply religious and strictly conservative. She met a boyfriend during her freshman year, and at the age of 17, she became pregnant because they did not use contraception. Because she was afraid of her parents, she decided to keep the information to herself at first. She also did not discuss this matter with her classmates due to shyness, which is a common cultural feeling among Filipinos. She did not visit a prenatal center to check on her condition. Her boyfriend, who is also a young man, decided not to face the consequences of their actions and advised her to just keep it a secret until she gives birth. Thus, Diva decided to keep her pregnancy a secret. No one knews about her situation, not even her teachers. She usually wears tighter clothes to school to cover her stomach, which is getting bigger. Until she had excessive bleeding one day and had to rush to the clinic after fainting in class. Then, she was checked by the physician and found out that she was pregnant. The case is called sudden infant death syndrome (SIDS), and she was fortunate to save herself, but her baby died. As a result, she suffers from severe depression and attempts suicide on several occasions. She had post-traumatic experiences as a result of what happened and regretted keeping the child for so long, holding herself solely responsible for the child's death. This event causes her to drop out of school and not complete her studies. She underwent several psychosocial counseling sessions.

A few years later, she found a new relationship with another guy, but the man took a video of their sexual encounter and shared it with his colleagues. As a result, she decided to seek the help of a social worker in filing a case and repeatedly blame herself for not being a virgin for the fact that this guy did not respect her. Although Philippine society is highly modernized there are still many men who preferred a relationship with someone who does not have prior sexual experiences. In addition, she did not finish her studies, so she was dependent on men for her economic source. The psychological repercussions of what happened to her in college were repeated. She felt revictimized and was referred for psychological evaluation, and her case was managed by a social worker using gender-responsive case management.

This study aims to provide a perspective on teen pregnancy that must be assessed from a gender perspective to see how our gender biases and stereotypes affect multiple factors in our society. A schematic diagram of how such factors intersect with gender issues and how we view women in our society is shown in the figure below.

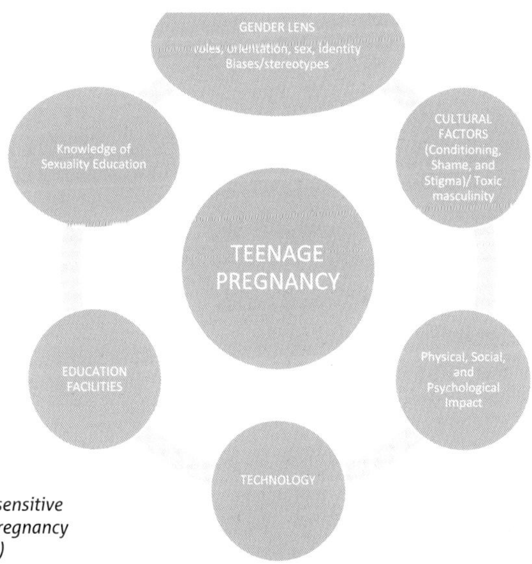

Figure 1. A gender-sensitive approach to early pregnancy (schematic diagram)

#08 Philippines
Analyzing Gender Aspects of Teenage Pregnancy in the Philippines

The diagram presented the importance of recognizing how the gender lens, which refers to how we view traditional roles, orientation, sexual identity, and biases and stereotypes of one's gender, affects how we see a situation like early pregnancy. The client grew up in a conservative family and was taught to be submissive, as evidenced by her relationship with the opposite sexes remains silent about her pregnancy, and even when the child dies, she solely blames herself for the situation as it was her only responsibility. victim blaming, which usually happens to women who experience abuse. They are passive-aggressive since this is also their coping mechanism for the problem presented to them. This silence will be reinforced by a culture that conditions people not to discuss private matters, like sexuality and pregnancy. the culture that attached shame and stigma to sensitive topics like sex at a young age. Teachers are the ones who provide education. Teachers must provide a gender-neutral environment for their students. Regardless of whether they are aware of it, they contribute to the gender gap in the classroom (Younger, Warrington, & Jacquetta, 1999). Her lack of education about sexuality is a sign that there is a knowledge gap that should be extensive for women like her to be protected from all forms of sexually transmitted diseases and unplanned pregnancies. Gender insensitivity affects the education industry (Orange, 2016). Many factors contribute to gender insensitivity, including fewer girls enrolling in school because of inadequate infrastructure. The school should provide adequate hygiene and sanitation facilities for both male and female students (Anita, Nargis, & Yasmin, 2010). D. Kalra, P. D. Research, and A. Sharma (2020) Another important consideration is the technology in our modern times, which may promote further violence against women, as this is also used by men to expose women's sexual activity without their consent, but only for their consumption, with the perspective that women are objects and subjects and not treated as persons with dignity. Canadian Journal of Disability Studies (n.d.) stated that technology is now being used by abusers to further these harms, whether it is intimate partner violence, gender-based harassment, hate campaigns, or misinformation campaigns (European Institute for Gender Equality 2017). By making it easier for abusers to access their targets, digital technologies have facilitated such forms of abusive behavior. The lack of comprehensive sex education remains a challenge for the Philippines in claiming to be a gender-fair society. These factors encountered by the client, in this case, may not be faced by males because they are excluded from these discussions in early pregnancy. The focus of schools is on young women who will become mothers, and if they are in this situation, schools will advise them to stop schooling and focus on giving birth, and some of them may not be able to come back and return to their studies because motherhood becomes their burden. Because of the gradual increase in gender-based violence in schools, it is critical to creating a gender-friendly environment. Gender sensitization in schools should be strengthened to help develop a gender-positive worldview and change how society perceives gender (Kalra & Sharma, 2019a). D. Kalra, P. D. Research, and A. Sharma (2020)

IMPLICATIONS TO STUDY. Various kinds of the literature revealed numerous reasons why teen pregnancy has become a problem in the Philippines, as well as how micro (individual), mezzo (school and family), and macro (such as poverty and technology) factors all contributed to the rising number of teen pregnancies. This leads to the conclusion that we lack a gender lens to examine the contribution of gender perspectives to these various factors and how they intersect remains a challenge in the context of education, health, and even technological aspects. Gender biases and stereotypes in different institutions in our society contributed to the problem of teenage pregnancy. If we see the value of gender sensitivity and gender analysis in understanding the problem then we can see the variety of gender issues and the gender gap in the context of this topic. The literature cited indicates that teen pregnancy can be prevented with the help of programs or elements that increase girls' self-esteem or confidence, as well as sexual and reproductive health education. Levtov, R. (2014) The evaluation of studies also showed that there is a lack of educational platforms that directly address the root causes of this gender concern. Moreover, pieces of literature show that young women's gender and sexuality education at home and in school is not fully operational. A safe space for discussions about women's hygiene, menstruation, gender, and sexuality in schools has not been fully explored by students and teachers. Although these are initiatives to teach about sex education, they do not directly address the root causes of the problem, which can be better understood if the problem is analyzed through a gender-sensitive lens. The United Nations Development Programme (UNDP) adopted the "2030 Agenda" with 17 Sustainable Development Goals in September 2015. (SDG). All of the objectives concern human lives and the environment. Goal number three is particularly pertinent to this study because it relates to ensuring that we live healthy lives and promote well-being for all ages. Furthermore, goal 3.7 states that by 2030, all countries must provide universal access to sexual and reproductive healthcare services, including family planning, education, and the incorporation of reproductive health into national strategies and programs (https://www.undp.org). The Philippines ranks 113th out of 189 countries on the Human Development Index (HDI), making it a medium-ranking country. Durrani, R., & Nielsen, A. (n.d.). In South Korea, a Gender and Sexuality Center was established to allow parents and children to communicate and discuss their sexuality and gender concerns at a young age. This type of opportunity allowed parents and children to actively share information about their children's physical and sexual development as they grew up. The center also promotes relevant gender-sensitive education through the creative methodology and the use of technology, and if parents and educators followed this mode, they could also instill Korean values in their children. Lack of such mechanisms in the Philippines and looking at the problem without finding more concrete mechanisms on how we should help young women and men not to engage in early pregnancy by providing them with appropriate education and interventions. The study implies engaging students, parents, and teachers in sessions that promote gender analysis and gender sensitivity and by consultation, they will be able to find ways to address the problem in more gender-fair strategies and interventions.—

REFERENCES

T. Libo-on, J., F. Manzo, J., & I. Manzo, O. (2021). Teenage Pregnancy: A Mother's Perspective. International Journal of Social Sciences Perspectives, 8(2), 50–55. https://doi.org/10.33094/7.2017.2021.82.50.55 • Adolescent and Youth Reproductive Health in the Philippines, Baccay, K.-L. B., Ngaya-An, F. v, & Marinduque, B. R. (n.d.). Predictors of Family Planning Practices of Teen Mothers in Manila, Philippines. Canadian Journal of Disability Studies. (n.d.). www.cjds.uwaterloo.ca • Capanzana, M. v., Aguila, D. v., Javier, C. A., Mendoza, T. S., & Santos-Abalos, V. M. (2015). Adolescent Pregnancy and the First 1000 Days (the Philippine Situation). Asia Pacific Journal of Clinical Nutrition, 24(4), 759–766. https://doi.org/10.6133/apjcn.2015.24.4.07 • Durrani, R., & Nielsen, A. (n.d.). "I've become hopeful again." A qualitative study of how the work of NGOs can be beneficial for teenage mothers in the Philippines. Galabo, N. R., & Gempes, G. P. (2017). Teenage Pregnancy in Secondary Schools: A Multiple Case Study. International Journal of Sciences: Basic and Applied Research (IJSBAR) International Journal of Sciences: Basic and Applied Research, 36(2), 145–170. http://gssrr.org/index.php?journal=JournalOfBasicAndApplied • Habito, C. M., Morgan, A., & Vaughan, C. (2021). Early union, 'disgrace', and prior adversity and disadvantage: pathways to adolescent pregnancy among Filipino youth. Reproductive Health, 18(1). https://doi.org/10.1186/s12978-021-01163-2 • Kalra, D., Research, P. D., & Sharma, A. (2020). 6969 | Divya Kalra Swivel Of Gender Sensitive Assortment: An Educational Model To Analyse Gender Sensitisation Swivel Of Gender Sensitive Assortment: An Educational Model To Analyse Gender Sensitisation. 19(4), 6969–6998. https://doi.org/10.17051/ilkonline.2020.04.765104 • Odhiambo, J. N. (2018). Exploring the Underlying Causes and Psychological Consequences of Teen Pregnancy in the Philippines (Vol. 21, Issue 2). Parungao, C. R., Bautista, L. P., Mariano, R., Bonifacio, V. M., & Aguinaldo, M. v. (2014). Life Brought at a Tender Age: The Lived Experiences of Filipino Teenage Pregnant Women. Asia Pacific Journal of Multidisciplinary Research, 2(1). www.apjmr.com • Ray, R., & Gatbonton, G. (n.d.). Educational Experiences of Adolescent Mothers while Studying College in the Philippines. In Philippines IAFOR Journal of Education: Inclusive Education (Vol. 9). Salvador, J. T., Sauce, B. R. J., Alvarez, M. O. C., & Rosario, A. B. (2016). The Phenomenon of Teenage Pregnancy in the Philippines. European Scientific Journal, ESJ, 12(32), 173. https://doi.org/10.19044/esj.2016.v12n32p173 • Sherpa, T. (n.d.). Factors Affecting Teenage Pregnancy in the Philippines. https://www.guttmacher.org/sites/default/files/report_p • Snyder, H. (2019). Literature review as a research methodology: An overview and guidelines. Journal of Business Research, 104, 333–339. https://doi.org/10.1016/j.

jbusres.2019.07.039 • Status, Issues, Policies, and Programs C. A. Varga Consultant I. Zosa-Feranil POLICY Project • Tabei, K., Cuisia-Cruz, E. S. S., Smith, C., & Seposo, X. (2021). Association between teenage pregnancy and family factors: An analysis of the philippine national demographic and health survey 2017. Healthcare (Switzerland), 9(12). https://doi.org/10.3390/healthcare9121720

AUTHOR

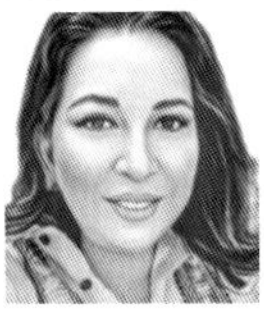

Amelyn L. Laro, RSW, MASW
Social Worker, ASIAN Gender Trainer/Community Solutions Fellow Gender, and Human Rights Research Fellow, International Sustainable Academy – +4915510554474 (Germany)
Social Work Faculty, Southern Philippines Agribusiness Marine and Aquatic School of Technology – Tel.+639055854297 / E-mail: Laro@ISA-Fellow@yahoo.com / Laro@Spamast.edu.ph, Amelyn Laro (researchgate.net)

isa. International Sustainability Academy

ISA is a project of the Schutzgemeinschaft Deutscher Wald Lv. Hamburg e.V. (SDW) [The Protective Association for the German Forest] is located in Hamburg in the WÄLDERHAUS. Our goal is to support and strengthen international cooperation in the implementation of Sustainable Development Goals (SDGs). The scholarship is sponsored by the Federal Ministry for Economic Cooperation and Development (BMZ) and is aimed at interested parties in emerging countries and economies on the Development Assistance Committee (DAC) list. The Schutzgemeinschaft Deutscher Wald Landesverband Hamburg e.V. (SDW), as a NUN-certified education center for sustainable development (BNE), heads the ISA which is responsible for the scholarship-holders. The program will be sponsored until the end of 2024. Seven rounds are planned from September 2019 to December 2024. The main aim of the ISA sponsorship is the international transfer of knowledge which helps the 13 scholarship-holders to further develop their existing special fields and/or existing projects in terms of Sustainable Development Goals (SDGs). Of particular importance and given priority are activities concerning climate protection and gender equality in their home countries. The primary objective is the distinguishable change in the home country through the continuation of the projects and/or the perspectives, solution approaches, and contacts acquired.

www.isa-germany.com

#09 Uganda
Health situation of LGTB in Uganda
Michael Shibale

The health situation of the lesbian, gay, bisexual and transgender (LGBT) community in Uganda has been a topic of concern for many years. Uganda has a reputation as one of the most anti-LGBT countries in the world, with homosexuality punishable by life imprisonment under the country's Penal Code.

The stigma and discrimination faced by LGBT persons in Uganda contribute to their poor health outcomes. There is little access to LGBT-friendly healthcare services, and many LGBT individuals avoid seeking medical care altogether for fear of being mistreated by medical professionals. This lack of access to healthcare services can have dire consequences for those living with HIV/AIDS or other chronic illnesses.

In addition to the lack of adequate healthcare facilities, there is a dearth of research into the health needs of LGBT persons in Uganda. Without adequate data, it is difficult for healthcare providers to develop effective interventions or for policymakers to craft evidence-based policies to meet the needs of the LGBT community.

The lack of access to healthcare services has a significant impact on the mental health of LGBT individuals in Uganda. The constant fear of violence, persecution and discrimination can lead to anxiety, depression and other mental health conditions. LGBT persons in Uganda often lack a support system and may struggle with feelings of isolation and loneliness.

The government of Uganda has repeatedly demonstrated its hostility towards the LGBT community, which has further exacerbated their health situation. For instance, there have been reports of forced anal examinations, harassment and arbitrary arrests of LGBT individuals by the police. Such actions further erode the trust between the LGBT community and the government, making it less likely that LGBT persons will seek medical attention.

Despite these challenges, there have been some efforts to improve the health situation of the LGBT community in Uganda. Pride Initiative for Eastern Region Uganda (PIERU) and other civil society groups have stepped in to provide health services and support to LGBT individuals. Some private hospitals and clinics have also created LGBT-friendly zones where individuals can receive medical care without fear of discrimination.

In conclusion, the health situation of the LGBT community in Uganda remains dire due to discrimination, stigma and limited access to healthcare services. In order to improve their health outcomes, there needs to be a concerted effort by healthcare providers, policymakers and civil society organizations to provide access to quality healthcare and support for LGBT individuals. At PIERU we want to set up a drop in center to solve some of these challenges.—

AUTHOR

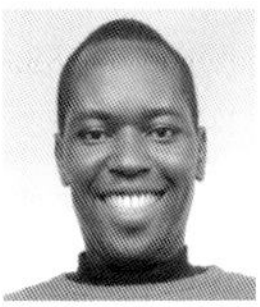

Michael Shibale
Pride Initiative for Eastern Region Uganda (PIERU)
ifa fellow 2023
pieru.uganda@gmail.com
https://pieruuganda.org/

PIERU
Pride Initiative for Eastern Region Uganda
HUMAN RIGHTS FOR ALL

#10.1 Ukraine

Ukrainian public health system's response to the challenges posed by the armed invasion of the Russian Federation in the territory of Ukraine

Hanna Saturska, Arkadii Shulhai, Nataliia Markiv-Bukovska, Nataliia Terenda, Nataliia Panchyshyn, Yurii Petrashyk

ABSTRACT. BACKGROUND. The armed invasion of the Russian Federation in the territory of Ukraine which escalated on February 24th 2022 has significantly increased the number of internally displaced persons in Ukraine and resulted in millions of Ukrainians fleeing their homeland to countries throughout Europe. The United Nations High Commissioner for Refugees currently estimates a total of 8,108,448 refugees. Many of them live or spend a certain amount of time in specially equipped places for IDPs/refugees. Large crowds in train cars and overnight accommodation, lack of sustainable access to running water and hygiene facilities can lead to outbreaks and rapid spread of infectious diseases. This had to be prevented using adequate prevention measures. These include ensuring a constant water supply, proper sanitation and access to medical services, as well as supervision and professional assistance from the CDC specialists.

THE PURPOSE OF THE STUDY: To study the response of the public health system to the challenges posed by the armed invasion of the Russian Federation in the territory of Ukraine, taking into account the experience and activities of the State Institutions: Ministry of Health of Ukraine, Public Health Centre of the Ministry of Health of Ukraine, Ternopil Regional Centre for Disease Control and Prevention of the Ministry of Health of Ukraine.

RESEARCH METHODS: scientific methods of systematic approach and systematic analysis were used to identify the features of the public health system in Ukraine in response to the challenges posed by the armed invasion of the Russian Federation in the territory of Ukraine.

RESULTS AND DISCUSSION. For the purpose of prevention of outbreaks and rapid spread of infectious diseases, adequate prevention measures had to be used in the public health system's response to the armed aggression of the Russian Federation against Ukraine, including ensuring constant water supply, proper sanitation and access to medical services provided by the Ministry of Health of Ukraine which had issued specific Orders. During the inspection (monitoring) of temporary accommodation facilities, the monitoring groups assessed the state of compliance with the Minimum Requirements for Ensuring Sanitary and Epidemiological

Welfare of the Population during the Emergency Arrangement of Temporary Accommodation Facilities for Internally Displaced Persons in connection with the armed aggression of the Russian Federation. The CDC specialists also carry out monitoring visits to places of temporary residence of internally displaced persons in order to ensure their right to live in a safe and healthy environment. This right is exercised by complying with the requirements for accommodation, food, water supply, laboratory control of food and drinking water, a set of preventive and anti-epidemic measures to prevent the introduction, occurrence and spread of infectious diseases among persons in places of temporary residence, as well as the provision of medical care, i.e. with the active participation of public health professionals.

CONCLUSIONS. The main task of the public health system now is to save the people of Ukraine from infectious diseases, outbreaks and epidemics and other consequences of Russia's disruptive invasion. Despite the fact that at the time of Russia's disruptive invasion, the main actors in the public health sector of Ukraine were in the process of transforming their functions and powers, and some were reorganizing, the public health system of Ukraine demonstrated a strong response to the challenges of wartime.

KEYWORDS. Public Health system, armed invasion of the Russian Federation in the territory of Ukraine.

INTRODUCTION. The armed aggression of the Russian Federation against Ukraine, which escalated on February 24th 2022, has significantly increased the number of internally displaced persons in Ukraine and resulted in millions of Ukrainians fleeing their homeland to countries throughout Europe. The United Nations High Commissioner for Refugees currently estimates a total of 8,108,448 refugees. Many of them live or spend a certain amount of time in specially equipped places for IDPs/refugees. Large crowds in train cars and overnight accommodation, lack of sustainable access to running water and hygiene facilities can lead to outbreaks and rapid spread of infectious diseases. This had to be prevented using adequate prevention measures. These include ensuring a constant water supply, proper sanitation and access to medical services, as well as supervision and professional assistance from the CDC specialists[1, 2].

THE PURPOSE OF THE STUDY: To study the response of the public health system to the challenges posed by the armed aggression of the Russian Federation against Ukraine, taking into account the experience and activities of the State Institutions "Ministry of Health of Ukraine", "Public Health Centre of the Ministry of Health Institutions: Ministry of Health of Ukraine,

#10.1 Ukraine
Ukrainian public health system's response to the challenges posed by the armed invasion of the Russian Federation in the territory of Ukraine

Public Health Centre of the Ministry of Health of Ukraine, Ternopil Regional Centre for Disease Control and Prevention of the Ministry of Health of Ukraine.

RESEARCH METHODS: scientific methods of systematic approach and systematic analysis had been used to identify the features of the public health system in Ukraine in response to the challenges posed by the armed aggression of the Russian Federation against Ukraine.

RESULTS AND DISCUSSION. For the purpose of prevention of outbreaks and rapid spread of infectious diseases, adequate prevention measures had to be used in the public health system's response to the armed aggression of the Russian Federation against Ukraine, including ensuring a constant water supply, proper sanitation and access to medical services provided by the Ministry of Health of Ukraine issued Order No. 584 of 06.04.2022 "On Approval of the Procedure for Conducting Surveys (Monitoring) in Places of Temporary Stay of Internally Displaced Persons in Connection with the armed aggressionof the Russian Federation". The survey (monitoring) is carried out in order to prevent the deterioration of the sanitary and epidemiological situation with regard to infectious diseases, including acute intestinal infectious diseases, and food poisoning among internally displaced persons in places of temporary stay[1].
In accordance with this order, the CDC specialists:

1) analyse the epidemiological situation in the region regarding infectious diseases, including acute intestinal infectious diseases, and food poisoning among internally displaced persons in places of temporary residence;
2) determine the list of places of temporary stay of increased epidemic risk for infectious diseases, including acute intestinal infectious diseases, and food poisoning;
3) based on the results of the analysis of the epidemic situation, draw up a regional plan for the inspection (monitoring) of places of temporary stay (hereinafter referred to as the plan), which is submitted for approval to the relevant regional, Kyiv city state administration (for the period of martial law – military administration);
4) inspect (monitor) places of temporary stay by monitoring groups, the composition of which is approved by the relevant order of the CCMC. Based on the results of the inspection (monitoring), an Act of Sanitary and Epidemiological Inspection of the facility is drawn up and submitted to the relevant Kyiv city or regional state administration (for the period of martial law – military administration)[1].
In accordance with this order, the specialists of the CDC:
1) analyse the epidemiological situation in the region regarding infectious diseases, including acute intestinal infectious diseases, and food poisoning among internally displaced persons in places of temporary stay;

2) determine the list of places of temporary stay of increased epidemic risk for infectious diseases, including acute intestinal infectious diseases, and food poisoning;
3) based on the results of the analysis of the epidemic situation, draw up a regional plan for the inspection (monitoring) of places of temporary stay (hereinafter referred to as the plan), which is submitted for approval to the relevant regional, Kyiv city state administration (for the period of martial law - military administration);
4) inspect (monitor) places of temporary stay by monitoring groups, the composition of which is approved by the relevant order of the CCMC. Based on the results of the inspection (monitoring), an Act of Sanitary and Epidemiological Inspection of the facility is drawn up and submitted to the relevant Kyiv city or regional state administration (for the period of martial law – military administration)[1].
During the inspection (monitoring) of temporary accommodation facilities, the monitoring groups assessed the state of compliance with the Minimum Requirements for Ensuring Sanitary and Epidemiological Welfare of the Population during the Emergency Arrangement of Temporary Accommodation Facilities for Internally Displaced Persons in connection with the Armed Aggression of the Russian Federation, approved by the Order of the Ministry of Health of Ukraine No. 458 of 10.03.2022, which expired on 22 April 2022 in accordance with the Order of the Ministry of Health of Ukraine No. 672.
The Ternopil Regional Centre of the Ministry of Health also demonstrated an appropriate level of response. Thus, pursuant to the Decree of the President of Ukraine of 24 February 2022 No. 64/2022, guided by Article 41 of the Law of Ukraine "On Ensuring Sanitary and Epidemic Welfare of the Population", the Regulation on the Functional Subsystem of Medical Protection of the Population, approved by the Order of the Ministry of Health of Ukraine of 25 March 2019 No. 667, the letter of the Ministry of Health of Ukraine of 24. 02.2022 No. 26-04/5359/2-22, on the first day of the armed aggression of the Russian Federation against Ukraine, the Director General issued an order "On the Formation and Functioning of Groups", according to which the following groups were formed:

I. directly at the Ternopil Regional Centre for the Prevention of HIV/AIDS:

1. Radiation monitoring and dosimetric control consisting of two teams;
2. Chemical monitoring and control consisting of two teams;
3. Epidemiological surveillance and control consisting of two teams.

II. In the Chortkiv City-District Centre of the MHC of Ukraine, the following were established:

1. A group of radiation monitoring and dosimetric control;

2. Chemical monitoring and control group;
3. Epidemiological surveillance and control group;
4. Disinfection team.

III. The Borshchiv Department of the Chortkiv City-District Centre of the Ministry of Health established the following:

1. Radiation monitoring and dosimetric control group;
2. Chemical monitoring and control group;
3. Epidemiological surveillance and control groups (main and reserve);
4. Disinfection teams (main and reserve);

IV. The Buchach department of the Chortkiv Interdistrict Centre of the Ministry of Health of Ukraine established the following:

1. A group of radiation monitoring and dosimetric control;
2. Chemical monitoring and control group;
3. Epidemiological surveillance and control group;
4. Disinfection team.

V. The Kremenets City-District Centre of the MHC of Ukraine established the following:

1. Radiation monitoring and dosimetric control group;
2. Chemical monitoring and control group;
3. Epidemiological surveillance and control group;
4. Disinfection team.

VI. In the Ternopil City-District Centre of the MHC of Ukraine, the following were established:

1. Chemical surveillance and control group;
2. An epidemiological surveillance and control group;
3. Disinfection team.

VII. The Koziv department of the Ternopil City-District Centre of the MHC of Ukraine established the following:

1. A group of radiation monitoring and dosimetric control;
2. Chemical monitoring and control group;
3. Epidemiological surveillance and control group;
4. Disinfection team.

VIII. The Terebovlya Department of the Ternopil City-District Centre of the MHC of Ukraine established the following:

1. A group of radiation monitoring and dosimetric control;
2. Chemical monitoring and control group;
3. Epidemiological surveillance and control group;
4. Disinfection team.

The above-mentioned order appointed a regional coordinator responsible for the activities of these groups.

Since the day of military aggression, the regional coordinator has performed the following functions:

1. Ensures daily monitoring in 24/7 mode.
2. Organises and controls the daily monitoring of the quality and safety of

drinking water supplied to the population in terms of microbiological, sanitary and chemical indicators in accordance with the rules "Hygienic requirements for drinking water intended for human consumption" (Sanitary and Epidemiological Requirements 2.2.4-171-10).

3. Ensures constant exchange of information with drinking water supply companies to obtain operational data on the state of water of surface and underground water sources, quality and safety of drinking water supplied to the water supply system (WSS).
4. Organises drinking water testing in healthcare facilities and other critical infrastructure facilities upon request from civil-military administrations.
5. Organise monitoring of gamma radiation at existing monitoring points with a frequency of at least 3 times per day.

In case of deviations based on the results of laboratory tests (within 2 hours), the Ministry of Health, the military-civilian administration, and the relevant communities are immediately informed.

Starting from 24.02.2022, the CPC immediately began to coordinate actions with the relevant territorial bodies of the SES to involve employees of the institution to conduct atmospheric air studies in the event of accidents at critical infrastructure facilities involving chemical agents.

The Department of Healthy Lifestyle Promotion of the CPC was authorised to inform the public about appropriate measures to be taken in case of abnormalities in the laboratory results.

The CDC specialists also carry out monitoring visits to places of temporary residence of internally displaced persons in order to ensure their right to live in a safe and healthy environment [3]. This right is exercised by complying with the requirements for accommodation, food, water supply, laboratory control of food and drinking water, a set of preventive and anti-epidemic measures to prevent the introduction, occurrence and spread of infectious diseases among persons in places of temporary residence, as well as the provision of medical care, i.e. with the active participation of public health professionals.

The CDC is responding to chemical threats in an appropriate manner. On 4 April, at 23.30, another air attack was carried out on the Ternopil region. The enemy missile missed its target and was shot down by air defence forces in the Kremenets district, but the debris fell on a mineral fertiliser warehouse and damaged six tanks. Immediately collected water samples showed elevated levels of ammonia in the soil and the Ikva River. Residents of the areas along the Ikva River in the Kremenets district were advised by the CCPC not to use water from wells for food. Fishing was prohibited. Experts of the Ternopil Regional

#10.1 Ukraine
Ukrainian public health system's response to the challenges posed by the armed invasion of the Russian Federation in the territory of Ukraine

Center for Chemical Control and Prevention of the Ministry of Health took water samples for ammonia content from 8 wells of private estates and two water towers in the village of Sapaniv, Kremenets district. Only two wells showed a slight excess of chemical compounds. In the others, the ammonia content was 0.05 mg/l, while the norm is 2.6 mg/l. The experts also examined a number of samples of the water supply network from the village's artesian wells, and the water met the standards. In addition, the Ternopil RECC staff took water samples from seven (7) points downstream of the Ikva River and monitored the water quality on a daily basis until all indicators were stabilized.

The CDC also proved to be excellent in the fight against particularly dangerous infections, including diphtheria. A 29-year-old resident of Sloviansk, who moved to Ternopil region, was confirmed to have diphtheria as of 31.03.2022. The woman was treated in Chortkiv hospital, there is no threat to her life. During the epidemiological investigation, specialists identified 70 contact persons at the place of residence (61 internally displaced persons and 9 employees of the institution) and treatment (9 persons). On 02.04.–03.04.2022, a bacteriological examination of all contact persons (79 persons in total) was carried out, the results of 06.04.–07.04.2022 were negative for Corynebacterium, and on 11.04.–12.04.2022, a bacteriological examination of contact persons (79 persons in total) was carried out, the results of 15.04.2022 were negative for Corynebacterium. Medical observation of the contacts was organised for 10 days (02.–11.04.2022), consultation with an ENT specialist, antibiotic prophylaxis, and vaccinations according to epidemiological indications. Antibiotics were prescribed for prophylactic purposes to 69 contacts, and 48 were vaccinated. The final disinfection was carried out in the outbreak (02.04.2022).

Prior to that, the last case of diphtheria in Ternopil region was registered in 2019. At that time, the disease was detected in a man who came from another region, and the last diagnosis among residents of Ternopil region was confirmed in 2012.

In accordance with the requirements of the current legislation, in order to ensure the sanitary and epidemiological well-being of the population during the elimination of the consequences of the armed aggression of the Russian Federation against Ukraine, the Ministry of Health issued Order No. 597 of 08.04.2022 "Some issues of ensuring the sanitary and epidemiological well-being of the population during the elimination of the consequences of the armed aggression of the Russian Federation against Ukraine" [4].

In accordance with this Order, the regional and Kyiv City Centralized Laboratory Centres of the Ministry of Health of

Ukraine, Zhytomyr Regional Laboratory and Laboratory Centres of the Ministry of Health of Ukraine on the territories of settlements temporarily occupied by the armed forces of the Russian Federation and where Ukraine's state sovereignty has been secured (restored), provided that there are no reports of possible radiation, chemical, biological and nuclear risks in the respective territories

1) ensure the study of the quality and safety of drinking water supplied to the population, including from non-centralised water supply sources, in terms of sanitary, chemical and microbiological indicators in accordance with the indicators specified in Annexes 1 and 2 to the State Sanitary Norms and Rules "Hygienic Requirements for Drinking Water Intended for Human Consumption" (DSanPiN 2.2.4-171-10), approved by the Order of the Ministry of Health of Ukraine No. 400 dated 12 May 2010, registered with the Ministry of Justice of Ukraine on 1 July 2010 under No. 452/17747. The location of the sampling points is determined in relation to the water supply scheme of the settlement and the characteristics of water intakes. Prior to receiving the results of laboratory tests, the centres recommended hyperchlorination of water in order to prevent outbreaks of infectious diseases associated with waterborne diseases;

2) ensure soil testing near (around) accident sites of chemical facilities, fuel and chemical storage facilities, and industrial enterprises. The scope, number of points and list of indicators are agreed with representatives of the SES territorial bodies, taking into account the actually destroyed infrastructure;

3) submit proposals to the regional, Kyiv city military administrations and local self-government bodies on the disinfestation of the territory of settlements and/or ensure that disinfection teams independently carry out the above measures, if they are involved;

4) submit proposals to the regional, Kyiv city military administrations and local self-government bodies on reburial of the remains of the deceased from mass and single burials located outside the territory of cemeteries and other burial sites;

5) recommend to the regional, Kyiv city military administrations and local self-government bodies to inspect mine wells, spring caps and pump rooms, repair, clean and disinfect them. In case the drinking water of mine wells, spring capsules and pump rooms does not meet the epidemic safety indicators, it is recommended to post an information sign "Water is not suitable for drinking" after the cleaning and disinfection measures and to carry out repeated cleaning and disinfection with further laboratory control of their effectiveness and public information. If involved, participate in the implementation of these measures;

6) ensure sanitary and epidemiological reconnaissance and prevention of infectious diseases, including typhoid and

typhoid fever, dysentery, tularemia, and other particularly dangerous infections;
7) ensure the indication and identification of pathogens of especially dangerous infections with the examination of environmental objects and differential diagnostic and research material from people with suspected especially dangerous infections (depending on the landscape of endemic diseases in a particular area);
8) submit proposals to the regional, Kyiv city military administrations and local self-government bodies on the sanitary cleaning of combat zones by means of rational sanitary cleaning of the combat zone with disinfection of human and animal corpses and other sanitary hazardous objects, removal and disinfection of sewage and other disinfection, disinsection and deratization measures in settlements, railway and road transport (if necessary);
9) in case of deviations from the results of laboratory tests, immediately (within 2 hours) inform the regional and Kyiv city military administration with proposals for appropriate response measures to ensure the sanitary and epidemiological well-being of the population, with further informing the state institution "Public Health Centre of the Ministry of Health of Ukraine" and the Ministry of Health of Ukraine about the measures taken;
10) ensure effective communication with the population on basic skills for the prevention of infectious diseases, peculiarities of water use (bottled water, the need for boiling, etc.), cooking in unsuitable conditions, use of personal protective equipment, unscheduled vaccination against hepatitis A, etc. [4]. For example, as of the 8th week of the war, the specialists of the Ternopil Regional Center for Chemical Hygiene and Epidemiology of the Ministry of Health prepared and posted more than 45 such information materials on the Centre's page on the social network FACEBOOK (META).
11) work together with representatives of veterinary medicine authorities on the need for oral vaccination against rabies in stray animals.

The CPH, among other things, was authorised to:

- to provide expert support in assessing the risk of an epidemic situation and taking appropriate response measures to ensure sanitary and epidemiological well-being in the territory;
- to develop and disseminate information materials for use to ensure effective communication with the population on behavior in case of hazards and threats to their health, taking into account the specificity of the impact of the hazard factor [4]. The CPH specialists prepared and posted 23 information materials on the following topics on the official website of the Ministry of Health in the section "For Citizens": "Methods of water disinfection", "Specialized psychiatric care during the

war", "HIV prevention during the war", "How to cope with stress during the war", "Explosive objects: a risk that can cost lives", "How to perform primary wound care", etc.[2].

Considerable attention was paid to ensuring the chemical security of the state. Thus, on 26 April 2022, the Cabinet of Ministers of Ukraine issued Order No. 314-r "On Approval of the Action Plan for the Implementation of the Concept for Improving the Level of Chemical Safety until 2026"[5].

This plan, among other things, provides for:

- Improving legislation on health protection from the negative impact of chemicals, including the development and submission to the CMU of a draft act on approval of guidelines for determining the hazard of chemicals based on the criterion of endocrine disruption;
- Organising a system of medical care in cases of violations of chemical safety and chemicals management requirements;
- Organisation of emergency medical care for the population in case of chemical poisoning at home;
- Improvement of the system of monitoring chemicals in environmental components, namely, development and submission to the Cabinet of Ministers of Ukraine of a draft act on the creation of a data bank on the potential threat of transboundary emergencies at chemically hazardous enterprises;
- Developing a mechanism for comprehensive assessment of the level of environmental pollution by chemicals;
- Development of a risk assessment system for the harmful effects of chemicals on the health of workers and the public;
- Strengthening human resources in the field of chemical safety and chemicals management;
- Improvement of educational programs for training of specialists by educational institutions to ensure the development of competence in the field of chemical safety management and chemicals management;
- Ensuring that chemical safety issues are studied during the advanced training of managers and specialists involved in production related to the use of chemical technologies that pose a chemical hazard;
- Consideration of chemical safety and chemical product management issues in the standards of higher and professional higher education in a number of specialities, including 229 Public Health[5].

Therefore, it should be noted that in such extremely difficult conditions of military aggression, the Regional Health Care Systems of Ukraine [6] the Public Health Center of the Ministry of Health of Ukraine [7] ensured the control and safety of food products and water [8] despite the period of transformation and reformation in in the field of public health[9]. In addition, taking into account the plan for achieving the SUSTAINABLE

#10.1 Ukraine
Ukrainian public health system's response to the challenges posed by the armed invasion of the Russian Federation in the territory of Ukraine

DEVELOPMENT GOALS [10] and with the help of international organizations, in particular WHO [11, 12], it was possible to implement effective protection of the population of Ukraine from the spread and outbreaks of infectious diseases and to continue the control of non-communicable diseases.

CONCLUSIONS. The main task of the public health system now is to save the people of Ukraine from infectious diseases, outbreaks and epidemics and other consequences of the Russian disruptive invasion. Despite the fact that at the time of the Russian disruptive invasion, the main actors in the public health sector of Ukraine were in the process of transforming their functions and powers, and some regional CDC were reorganizing, the public health system of Ukraine demonstrated a strong response to the challenges of wartime.—

REFERENCES

1 [Order of the Ministry of Health "On Approval of the Procedure for Conducting Examination (Monitoring) in Places of Temporary Stay of Internally Displaced Persons in Connection with the Armed Aggression of the Russian Federation" 06.04.2022 No 584.] in Ukrainian [cited 2023 April 04]. Available at: https://zakon.rada.gov.ua/laws/show/z0408-22#Text **2** [Ministry of Health of Ukraine. Section "To the public"] in Ukrainian [cited 2023 April 04]. Available at: https://moz.gov.ua/gromadjanam **3** United Nations. General Assembly: 217 A (III). Universal Declaration of Human Rights. [cited 2023 April 04]. Available at: http://www.un-documents.net/a3r217a.htm **4** [Order of the Ministry of Health of Ukraine „Some Issues of Ensuring Sanitary and Epidemiological Welfare of the Population during the Elimination of the Consequences of the Armed Aggression of the Russian Federation against Ukraine" 08.04.2022 No 597.] in Ukrainian [cited 2023 April 04]. Available at: https://zakon.rada.gov.ua/rada/show/v0597282-22#Text **5** [Order of the Cabinet of Ministers of Ukraine "On Approval of the Action Plan for Implementation of the Concept of Chemical Safety Improvement until 2026" 26.04.2022 No 314.] in Ukrainian [cited 2023 April 04]. Available at: https://www.kmu.gov.ua/npas/pro-zatverdzhennya-planu-zahodiv-z-realizaciyi-koncepciyi-pidvishchennya-rivnya-himichnoyi-bezpeki-do-2026-roku-314-260422 **6** [Regional Public Health Systems. Public Health Centre of the Ministry of Health of Ukraine] in Ukrainian [cited 2023 April 04]. Available at: https://phc.org.ua/regionalni-cgz. **7** [Public Health Center of the Ministry of Health of Ukraine] in Ukrainian [cited 2023 April 04]. Available at: https://phc.org.ua/pro-centr/ustanovchi-dokumenti **8** CDC and Food Safety [cited 2023 April 04]. Available at: https://www.cdc.gov/foodsafety/cdc-and-food-safety.html **9** Public Health In Ukraine. Saturska H, Shulhai A, Terenda N, Panchyshyn N. Akkon Schriftenreihe Band 5. Public Health in Ukraine. Akkon Hochschule für Humanwissenschaften / Institute for Research in International Assistance (IRIA). September 2021. Pp. 12-18. [cited 2023 April 04]. Available at: https://www.akkon-hochschule.de/files/akkon/downloads/publikationen/5_Public%20Health%20in%20Ukraine.pdf **10** UNDP IN UKRAINE. SUSTAINABLE DEVELOPMENT GOALS. [cited 2023 April 04]. Available at: https://ukraine.un.org/en/sdgs **11** WHO, International Health Regulations. [cited 2023 April 04]. Available at: https://www.who.int/health-topics/international-health-regulations#tab=tab_1 **12** World Health Organization. STEPwise Approach to NCD Risk Factor Surveillance (STEPS) [cited 2023 April 04]. Available at: https://www.who.int/teams/noncommunicable-diseases/surveillance/systems-tools/steps

AUTHORS

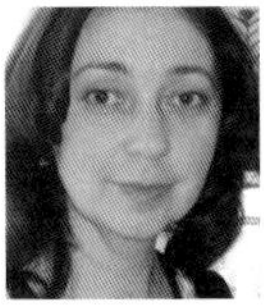

Prof., MD, DMSc, Hanna Saturska
Ivan Horbachevsky Ternopil National Medical University
2 Slovatskyi Street, 46000 Ternopil, Ukraine
Tel. +380980651672, saturska@tdmu.edu.ua

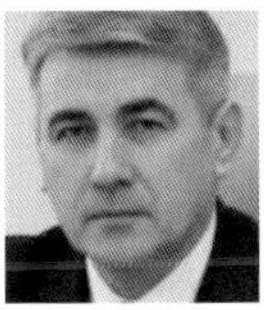

Prof., MD, DMSc, Arkadii Shulhai
Ivan Horbachevsky Ternopil National Medical University
2 Slovatskyi Street, 46000 Ternopil, Ukraine
Tel. +38 0352 525588, shulgai@tdmu.edu.ua

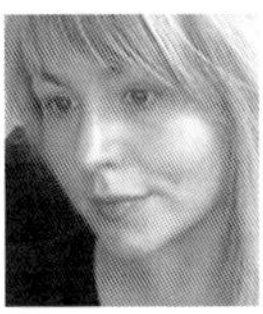

Natalia Markiv-Bukovska
State Institution "Ternopil Oblast Center for Diseases Control and Prevention of the Ministry of Health of Ukraine"
21A Kniazia Ostrozkoho Street, 46001 Ternopil, Ukraine
Tel. +380685150266, totemnb@gmail.com

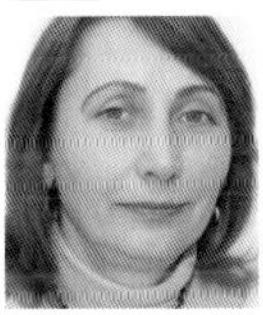

Prof., MD, DMSc, Nataliia Terenda
Ivan Horbachevsky Ternopil National Medical University
2 Slovatskyi Street, 46000 Ternopil, Ukraine
Tel. +380988020038, lisovska@tdmu.edu.ua

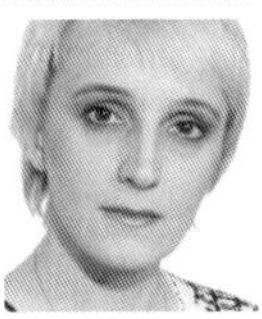

Assoc. Prof., MD, PhD, Nataliia Panchyshyn
Ivan Horbachevsky Ternopil National Medical University
2 Slovatskyi Street, 46000 Ternopil, Ukraine
Tel. +380970589389, panchyshyn@tdmu.edu.ua

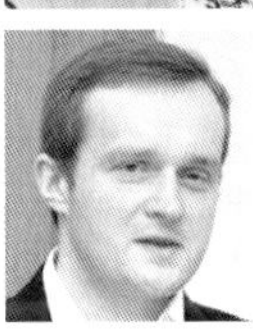

Yurii Petrashyk, PhD, MBA, Assoc. Prof.
Ivan Horbachevsky Ternopil National Medical University
2 Slovatskyi Street, 46000 Ternopil, Ukraine
Tel. +380673392342, yurii.m.petrashyk@tdmu.edu.ua

#10.2 Ukraine
The role of Public Health Centers in the prevention of eating disorders – example Ukraine

Diana Saturska, Ostap Saturskyi

OBJECTIVE – to determine the role of public health centers in the formation of proper nutrition principles in Ukraine at the current stage of development of public health system in the framework of achieving the Sustainable Development Goals.

MATERIALS AND METHODS. The analysis of available information resources of the Internet, foreign professional publications, and medical database MEDLINE/PubMed for the last five years is carried out. The method of information search and analytical-comparative method is applied.

RESULTS. Central and regional Centers for Disease Control and Prevention and Public Health Centers should take into account primarily the etiology of eating disorders, which today is quite heterogeneous, including biological, psychological, related to personality development and socio-cultural aspects. When studying the role of public health centers in Ukraine in the formation of proper eating behavior and nutrition principles, attention should be paid to the possibilities of solving this problem in Ukraine. However, not all public health centers in Ukraine contain such information that needs to be improved. It is important to pay attention to the fact that the information is presented correctly, taking into account the age, preferences, educational level of the population who will use this information most often.

CONCLUSIONS. Thus, for the prevention of eating disorders and achieving good nutrition of population in Ukraine at the present stage of development of public health system, among the many tools available for implementation by public health centers and centers for disease control and prevention the most effective ones are following: formation the positive attitude towards healthy lifestyle, formation of objective perception of one's own body, popularization of the correct principles of food culture in society and regular monitoring of food quality, taking into account the world experience of the centers for disease control and prevention in solving this problem.

KEY WORDS: centers for disease control and prevention, public health centers, nutrition, eating disorders.

INTRODUCTION. New challenges that have inevitably arisen before specialists in the field of health care and the public health system in Ukraine [2, 12] and on a global scale [14, 15, 16] necessitate the need for further improvement of the training of public health specialists and ensuring that they acquire the necessary professional competences for solving problems in the field of public health [5, 8], especially problems related to the nutrition of the population of different age groups and various nutritional disorders [7, 10, 13] that arise under the influence of stress factors and socio-economic determinants of health.

Nutrition is an important part of human health and development [5, 16]. Better nutrition improves the health of adults and children, especially infants, children and mothers, strengthens the immune system, contributes to the safe course of pregnancy and childbirth, reduces the risk of non-communicable diseases, in particular such as diabetes and cardiovascular diseases, contributes to active longevity and ensures a high quality of life for people of any age [14].

Scientists have proven that healthy children learn better and develop physically and spiritually. People with sufficient nutrition are more capable and productive, they are able to create greater opportunities for the development of society, the achievement of the Sustainable Development Goals and the gradual breaking of the cycles of poverty and hunger [13]. After all, one of the Sustainable Development Goals is Goal 2.2 "End all forms of malnutrition", including the achievement by 2025 of internationally agreed goals on stunting and wasting in children under the age of 5, as well as meeting the nutritional needs of adolescent girls, pregnant women and women, who feed babies and the elderly.

Malnutrition in any form poses a significant threat to human health. Today, the world faces the double burden of malnutrition, which includes both undernutrition and overweight, especially in low- and middle-income countries.

Among the problems associated with lack of nutrition and improper eating habits, eating disorders [7, 10], which are associated with psychological factors [6, 9], occupy a prominent place and can be a real threat to human life. In the conditions of rapid negative changes in people's lives, the effects of acute and chronic stress, this problem has become widespread in Ukraine and in all countries of the world. However, with proper and timely treatment, as well as with professional support, full recovery of such patients is possible.

Unfortunately, due to existing biases and prejudices about what people with eating disorders look like [3, 11], many of them do not seek the qualified help they need in time.

Eating disorders, such as anorexia nervosa, bulimia nervosa, and compulsive overeating, are currently an extremely urgent problem, as they are associated with significant negative medical and social consequences and have the highest mortality rate among all mental illnesses. Today, every 62 minutes at least one person dies from the effects of an eating disorder.

#10.2 Ukraine
The role of Public Health Centers in the prevention of eating disorders – example Ukraine

Eating disorders [7, 8, 10] can have serious consequences for the physical health, psychological and social well-being of adolescents, young people and adults, so it is extremely important to ensure their timely detection and seeking professional help. Even more important is the establishment of preventive mechanisms [4] to prevent these disorders, especially among adolescents and young people. In this aspect, an important role belongs to public health centers, or so-called disease control and prevention centers [2, 5, 12]. Currently, not only doctors, but also masters of public health solve complex complex tasks and problems, and ensure their solution, often with the involvement of interdisciplinary connections between various specialists, organizations and institutions. Therefore, clarifying the role of disease control and prevention centers and the public health center in solving nutrition problems and preventing eating disorders [4] is a priority direction of scientific research in the field of public health.

OBJECTIVE – to determine the role of public health centers in the formation of proper nutrition principles in Ukraine at the current stage of development of public health system in the framework of achieving the Sustainable Development Goals.

MATERIALS AND METHODS. The analysis of available information resources of the Internet, foreign professional publications, and medical database MEDLINE/PubMed for the last five years is carried out. The method of information search and analytical-comparative method is applied.

RESULTS AND DISCUSSION. According to the results of scientific research, every fifth death on our planet is caused by improper nutrition, namely diseases for which improper nutrition is the main risk factor [8, 10].
Among such diseases, the most common are diseases of the cardiovascular system, in particular, hypertension, heart attack, atherosclerosis, type II diabetes and malignant neoplasms, etc. Eating disorders are a group of psychogenic behavioral syndromes characterized by severe and persistent eating disorders, associated with disturbing thoughts and emotions. These can be very serious conditions that affect physical, psychological and social function.
Types of eating disorders include anorexia nervosa, bulimia nervosa, binge eating disorder, selective eating disorder and others. Selective eating disorder, is a condition in which people restrict the amount or type of food they eat. Unlike anorexia nervosa, people with binge eating disorder do not have a distorted body image or an extreme fear of gaining weight. This disorder is most common in childhood and usually has an earlier onset than other eating disorders.

Many children go through phases of picky eating. A child with selective eating disorder does not consume enough calories to grow and develop properly, and an adult does not consume enough calories to support basic body functions.

In general, eating disorders affect up to 5% of the population, most often develop in adolescence and young adulthood. Some, especially anorexia nervosa and bulimia nervosa, are more common among women, but all can occur at any age and affect either gender.

Eating disorders are often associated with excessive attention to food, weight, and body shape [3, 9, 11]. People with eating disorders often experience anxiety when thinking about and eating food. Behaviors associated with eating disorders, including restricting or avoiding certain foods, binge eating, purging (vomiting), abusing laxatives, or compulsive sport exercise. Such behavior often turns into psychological dependence on one's own obsessions.

Central and regional centers for disease control and prevention and public health centers [2, 5, 8] in the issues of solving nutrition problems and prevention of eating disorders should first of all take into account the etiology of eating disorders, which is currently quite heterogeneous, including biological, psychological, personality development and socio-cultural aspects.

Among socio-cultural factors, influences such as the popularization of thinness in society, the influence of a culture that values thin bodies for women and men, and the influence of media that promote such ideas play an important role in increasing the prevalence of eating disorders worldwide.

One in eight teenagers by the age of twenty may have at least one eating disorder. Every year, about 500,000 Ukrainians suffer from eating disorders. Although eating disorders can affect people of all ages and both sexes, they are most common in teenagers and young women. Anorexia nervosa and bulimia nervosa account for approximately 0.3% and 1% of adolescent girls, respectively. The prevalence of eating disorders tends to be higher in young women, with the exception of binge eating, which is more common in men and the elderly.

However, it should be remembered that some diseases can mimic eating disorders. Chronic infectious diseases, malabsorption, malignancy, immunodeficiency, endocrine disorders such as diabetes, hyperthyroidism or Addison's disease, which should be excluded before being labeled as an eating disorder. A strong fear of gaining weight and disfiguring one's body will be a characteristic feature of eating disorders, which will help exclude the other diseases mentioned above.

To study the influence of public health centers on the formation of the principles of proper eating behavior, the materials

#10.2 Ukraine
The role of Public Health Centers in the prevention of eating disorders – example Ukraine

posted on the official websites of regional public health centers in Ukraine and the world were analyzed [2, 5, 8].

The application of an integrated approach, the use of various data sources, both state statistical observation data and administrative data, provides a basis for an objective factual analysis, in accordance with international standards (evidence based analysis).

To monitor this problem, indicators are used, data according to which are collected and developed on an ongoing basis within the framework of the official statistical system, in accordance with established standards and methodologies, and administrative reporting of ministries, other central and local executive bodies, institutions, and organizations.

When studying the role of public health centers in Ukraine in forming the foundations and principles of proper eating behavior and rational nutrition in general, attention to the possibilities of solving this problem in Ukraine within the framework of achieving the Sustainable Development Goals was paid.

However, not all public health centers in Ukraine contain necessary information so it requires improvement.

It is important to take into consideration the fact that the information should be presented correctly, taking into account the age, preferences, educational level of the population that will most often use this information.

Accustoming to proper nutrition in schools is also very important. For this, specialists of the Ministry of Health of Ukraine developed special nutrition programs in educational institutions and children's health and resorts [1]. The following principles recommended by specialists of the Ministry of Health of Ukraine should be followed:

1. The energy and nutritional value of food (macro- and micronutrient content) in preschool, general secondary education institutions and other educational institutions that conduct educational activities at a certain level (levels) of full general secondary education, children's rehabilitation and recreation institutions must meet the general age needs of the students of education/children in accordance with the norms of physiological needs for basic nutrients and energy, determined by the Ministry of Health of Ukraine.
2. Planning the part of caloric content of food in total energy needs depends on the regime (multiplicity) of food in the institution.
3. If only breakfast is consumed, the caloric content should be 25–30% of the daily requirement, the corresponding portion for lunch increases to 30–35%.

Meat, fish, milk and dairy products, eggs, legumes and nuts are the main sources of protein. An additional source of useful proteins are cereals, grains, and legumes.

At least two-thirds of the fat consumed by learners/children should come as unsaturated fat (unsaturated fatty acids). Unsaturated fats include essential fatty acids and fat-soluble vitamins, so their consumption is mandatory for the proper structural and functional state of the body and its organs and systems, including the brain, nervous system, heart, blood vessels, endocrine system, vision, skin and hair . The intake of saturated fats should be limited to no more than 10 percent of the total daily caloric content and the caloric content of individual dishes. Reducing the consumption of saturated fats, mainly of animal origin, is associated with a reduction in the risk of diseases of the circulatory system.

It is recommended to replace saturated fats of animal origin with unsaturated fats of plant origin and regular presence of marine fish in dishes.

The content of sugars in food products intended for sale in buffets, vending machines offered to learners/children in institutions and in food products used for the preparation of ready meals is limited to a level of no more than 10 g per 100 g/ml of food product .

Food products intended for sale in buffets, vending machines, and meals offered to students/children in institutions must be without the addition of sweeteners, synthetic colors and flavors (except vanillin, ethyl vanillin and vanilla extract), flavor and aroma enhancers.

Parental influence on food preferences begins with decisions, however parents are limited by social influences, their own food choices, breastfeeding and how they feed their children.

Measures to educate parents about proper, rational nutrition for children are promising. Recommended parenting strategies to increase vegetable intake in early childhood include modeling, and encouraging trying with non-food rewards. Educational and preventive measures carried out in early childhood correspond to the time for the formation of food preferences, are, as a rule, more effective than measures with older children [14, 16].

Improper nutrition from early childhood affects the development of health problems and gaining excess body weight. In adolescence, children begin to evaluate themselves as individuals, and pay considerable attention to their appearance. It is in the puberty period that eating disorders usually begin to appear, so the basis of proper nutrition from an early age can serve as a method of primary prevention of this group of diseases.

CONCLUSIONS. Thus, for the prevention of eating disorders and rational nutrition in Ukraine at the current stage of development of the field of public health, among the many means available for implementation by public health centers and disease control and prevention centers, the most effective is the formation of a positive attitude among young people towards healthy lifestyle, forming an objective perception of one's own body, popularizing the correct principles of nutrition culture in society and regular monitoring of the quality of food products within the framework of achieving the Sustainable Development Goals. These measures should be carried out taking into account the global experience of the Centers for Disease Control and Prevention in solving this problem.

PROSPECTS FOR FURTHER RESEARCH consist in studying the effectiveness of various measures for the prevention of eating disorders and ensuring the rational nutrition of the population, implemented by public health centers and disease control and prevention centers.—

REFERENCES

1 The Verkhovna Rada of Ukraine "On the approval of norms and the Procedure for the organization of meals in educational institutions and children's health and recreation institutions" Available at: https://zakon.rada.gov.ua/laws/show/305-2021-%D0%BF#Text **2** Public Health Center of the Ministry of Health of Ukraine. Available at: https://phc.org.ua/pro-centr/ustanovchi-dokumenti **3** Associations of weight- or shape-related bullying with diverse disordered eating behaviors in adolescents. / Day S, Bussey K, Trompeter N, et al. // Int J Eat Disord. 2021 Sep;54(9):1641-1651. doi: 10.1002/eat.23573. Epub 2021 Jun 28. PMID: 34181288. **4** Bauer S. Prevention of eating disorder: a review / Bauer S., Kindermann S.S., Moessner M.Z // Kinder Jugendpsychiatr Psychother. 2017 Sep;45(5):403-413. doi: 10.1024/1422-4917/a000506. Epub 2016 Dec 13. PMID: 27951744. **5** CDC and Food Safety Available at: https://www.cdc.gov/foodsafety/cdc-and-food-safety.html **6** Discrimination and Eating Disorder Psychopathology: A Meta-Analysis. / Mason TB, Mozdzierz P, Wang S, Smith KE. // Behav Ther. 2021 Mar;52(2):406-417. doi: 10.1016/j.beth.2020.05.003. Epub 2020 May 30. PMID: 33622509. **7** Eating disorders as a public health issue: prevalence and attributable impairment of quality of life in an Italian community sample. / Carta MG, Preti A, Moro MF, et al. // International Review of Psychiatry, 2014 Aug;26(4):486-92. doi: 10.3109/09540261.2014.927753. PMID: 25137115. **8** Gaffney T. A decade without data eating disorder researchers say a gap in CDC survey has left them flying blind.. Available at: https://www.statnews.com/2021/12/09/eating-disorders-research-health-cdc/ **9** Is Cybervictimization Associated with Body Dissatisfaction, Depression, and Eating Disorder Psychopathology? / Marco JH, Tormo-Irun MP, Galán-Escalante A, et al. // Cyberpsychol Behav Soc Netw. – 2018 Oct;21(10):611-617. doi: 10.1089/cyber.2018.0217. PMID: 30334649. **10** NIMH: Eating Disorders. Available at: https://www.nimh.nih.gov/health/topics/eating-disorders **11** Policy Actions to Address Weight-Based Bullying and Eating Disorders in Schools: Views of Teachers and School Administrators. / Puhl RM, Neumark-Sztainer D, Bryn Austin S, et al. // J Sch Health. 2016 Jul;86(7):507-15. doi: 10.1111/josh.12401. PMID: 27246675. **12** Public Health In Ukraine. Saturska H, Shulhai A, Terenda N, Panchyshyn N. Akkon Schriftenreihe Band 5. Public Health in Ukraine. Akkon Hochschule für Humanwissenschaften / Institute for Research in International Assistance (IRIA). September 2021. Pp. 12-18. Available at: https://www.akkon-hochschule.de/files/akkon/downloads/publikationen/5_Public%20Health%20in%20Ukraine.pdf **13** UNDP IN UKRAINE. SUSTAINABLE DEVELOPMENT GOALS. Available at: https://www.ua.undp.org/content/ukraine/en/home/sustainable-development-goals.html **14** WHO: Comprehensive implementation plan on maternal, infant and young child nutrition. Available at: https://www.who.int/publications/i/item/WHO-NMH-NHD-14.1 **15** WHO: Healthy diet. Available at: https://www.who.int/news-room/fact-sheets/detail/healthy-diet **16** WHO: Recommendations on the marketing of foods and non-alcoholic beverages to children. Available at: https://www.who.int/publications/i/item/9789241500210

AUTHORS

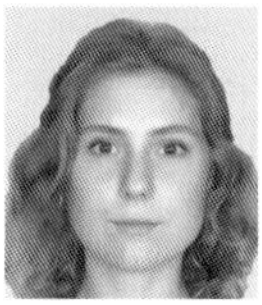

Diana Saturska
Ivan Horbachevsky Ternopil National Medical University
2 Slovatskyi Street, 46000 Ternopil, Ukraine
Tel.: +380933651357 | kollinsdiana1302@gmail.com

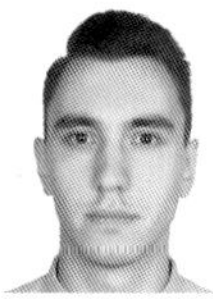

Ostap Saturskyi
Ivan Horbachevsky Ternopil National Medical University
2 Slovatskyi Street, 46000 Ternopil, Ukraine
Tel.: +380980267025 | saturskij.ov@gmail.com

#11 Yemen
Finding a Low-cost Substitute for Harmful Solid Waste Management Practices to Mitigate Health Risks in Yemen
Alaaddin Alqadsi

INTRODUCTION. When the war started in 2015, consequently, several governmental sectors in Yemen collapsed including the solid waste management (SWM) system. Government has very low capacities to handle solid waste in the entire country and in the rural areas specifically. Low capacities to handle solid waste in Yemen existed prior to the war. A (SWEEP-Net 2014) study mentioned that Municipal Solid waste (MSW) generation per capita in Yemen is 0.6 kg/day (urban areas) and 0.35 kg/day (rural areas) with annual 3% MSW generation growth rate.

Since 2015, the SWM system in Yemen has faced obstacles due to the ongoing war. The civil strife in 2011 led to a deadlock in institution and a halt in funding from international donors for SWM's national strategy. Importing restrictions have affected the availability of food, fuel, and the operation of machinery, impacting MSW generation rates. Air-strikes by the Saudi-led coalition have damaged SWM vehicles and tools, hindering access to SWM operations. The concentration of IDPs has led to a massive generation and disposal of solid waste in rural areas with low operation. The government's financial capacity has been reduced due to lower revenue and collected tax, resulting in the deterioration of major public services. (Olmo Forni et al. 2015)

THE ADOPTION OF HARMFUL SWM PRACTICES. Rural population has adopted wrong waste disposal practices as a result to the failure of government to manage solid waste. A baseline report of the 'CDH' Project showed the 70% of the surveyed population are burning their solid waste and 13% are disposing their solid waste in open areas. (YAQHSD 2022)

Households in some areas burn solid waste in an area near their dwelling, creating toxic fumes and hazards from glass and metal. Fires are difficult to control and cause inconvenience from constant smoke inhalation. Lack of transportation and equipment means waste is burned close to homes, increasing risks. This contributes to climate change due to increased CO2 emissions. (Humanitatian Innovation Fund 2016)

Disposing in open areas is another common practice, HHs in villages sometimes dispose solid waste in communal open areas that is identified or informally known to dispose the solid waste. These areas can vary in distance based on the arrangement of houses but mostly within less than 100m away from the dwellings. Usually, the disposal to the areas continues for a long period of time and then eventually being burnt. Same health risks as mentioned above are present. However, increased times of disposal with no action can intensify the health risk by giving more time for the flies to breed. In rainy seasons, the water collected in empty disposed containers encourages mosquito breeding. It is generally known that the distance between the land and the dwelling is directly proportional to the solid waste burning time. In some areas, the solid waste is never burnt and keeps accumulating forming pools of solid waste exposing the communities to extreme health risks and jeopardizing the quality of groundwater. (Humanitatian Innovation Fund 2016)

SOLID WASTE DISPOSAL OPTIONS. The Three feasible solution for solid waste management in rural areas could be sanitary landfills, communal pits, or family pits. Each one has its own advantages and disadvantages in terms of initial capital, operation, and maintenance.

a. Sanitary Landfills:

Sanitary landfills are an effective way to dispose of waste in emergency situations, reducing public health and environmental hazards. However, the process requires significant operational and financial capacity, including transportation of waste and substantial initial capital investment. Ongoing costs for salaries, fuel, and maintenance also require sustained funding (Humanitatian Innovation Fund 2016)

b. Communal Pits:

Direct waste disposal into a common pit is the most basic form of solid waste management. The number of individuals it serves will determine the size of this pit. Six cubic meters per fifty individuals is the suggested long-term goal. To reduce flies and other pests, waste should be covered with a thin layer of soil at least once every week. Such a system is rapid to implement and requires little operation and maintenance. The initial investment is low compared to the sanitary landfill option. (Humanitatian Innovation Fund 2016)

Households must transport solid waste to communal pits, which can be inconvenient if the distance is far. However, this method is simpler than transporting waste to sanitary landfills. A worker is needed for maintenance, but community-based or voluntary solutions are possible. During heavy rains, improper drainage can lead to groundwater contamination, so the location of pits relative to water sources is important . (Humanitatian Innovation Fund 2016)

c. Family Pits:

Where there is enough land, family pits might be a better long-term solution. Families should be urged to frequently cover waste with soil from sweeping or ash from cooking fires. These should be shallow (up to 1 m deep).

It is rapid to implement; and requires little operation and maintenance. Families are responsible for managing their own waste; no external waste workers are required. Low financial investment needed compared to the sanitary landfills. Community mobilization can be incorporated into hygiene promotion program.

RECYCLING. Most recycling is done through the informal sector and waste picking. Formal recycling of waste is an ideal practice to encourage as it is environmentally friendly and reduces the volume of landfill needed. However, because of the high level of organization and manpower needed, recycling is unlikely to be practicable in many emergency situations. Nevertheless, in the context of emergency, a certain amount of informal recycling is likely to occur, as there may be a shortage of items such as containers, bags, and other materials (Humanitatian Innovation Fund 2016).
Potential recycling models for the context in Yemen were discussed with representatives from the International Sustainability Academy (ISA). One of the most interesting models discussed was the "Trash for Cash" model implemented by a social enterprise in Nigeria. This model provides financial incentives for HH to encourage them in recycling their garbage at household level. For this, waste collection centers are established in the participating villages. At the collection centers, which are called "trash banks", HHs trade the recyclable materials (trash) for money, and thus have access to a source of an extra income. The collected materials are then transferred by workers to aggregation center and sold to local factories for further use or exported internationally.
The model could be applied to Yemen. However, modifications are necessary to ensure smooth operation of the model and to ensure its alignment with the work of non-for-profit organizations.

Cash for Trash original model vs Tailored Model

Step	Original Model	Tailored Model (Yemen)
1	**Trash sorting at HH level**	**Trash sorting at HH level** - Same as original model **Financial sustainability** A design of a business model to establish a self-sustained center
2	**Establishment of collection centers** **The social enterprise bares the cost of initiating the center**	**Establishment of collection centers** funded through grants/loans given to a person or a group of people as a part of livelihoods project.
3	**Hiring collection center staff**	Hiring collection center staff
4	**Establishment of aggregation centers** **aggregate the recyclable materials form different villages.**	**Linkage of collection centers to established businesses.** Not aggregation centers. However, Linkage to established business at district level. Materials will be sold to other businesses. The established businesses have already a network of contacts to deal with waste.
5	**Transportation to factories or export internationally**	Not Applicable

DISCUSSION. This article discussed common practices of waste disposal in Yemen, which can cause harm to the population and environment and shed light on possible alternatives.

As stated above, the feasibility of these alternatives depends on a lot of factors such as, financial and human resources, operation , and maintenance needs. Analyzing these factors and bearing in mind the situation in the targeted villages, we see two feasible approaches. For communal pits, minimum operation and maintenance might be required from the community which must coordinated among them.

On the other hand, the family pits can be fully dependent on the family that uses it and its operation and maintenance must be carried by the HH. In general, both solutions need minimum operation and maintenance. Thus, both, the communal and family pits, can be used alternatively in different villages based on the available space and the communities' readiness to participate in the operation.

"After 8 years of conflict, Yemenis face ongoing economic crisis, disrupted public services, and armed violence. An estimated 21.6 million people will require humanitarian assistance and protection services in 2023. Public services and infrastructure have been severely affected, and over 80% of the population struggles to access basic necessities such as food, safe drinking water, and healthcare. Almost 90% of Yemenis lack access to publicly supplied electricity. Additionally, public sector employees, including healthcare workers and teachers, have not received regular salaries in years." (Humanitarian Programme Cycle 2022)—

REFERENCES

Humanitarian Programme Cycle (2022): HUMANITARIAN NEEDS OVERVIEW YEMEN 2023. OCHA. • Humanitatian Innovation Fund (2016): WASH in Emergencies | Problem Exploration Report | Solid Waste Management. • Olmo Forni; Aiden Short, Ben Grundy; Martın Bjerregaard; Ramy Salemdeeb (2015): Emergency Waste Assessment in Yemen. • SWEEP-Net (2014): Country report on the solid waste management in YEMEN. • YAQHSD (2022): Baseline Report. Health Prevention through Capacity Development and Hygiene Measures in Yemen.

[i]The project full name is "Health Prevention through Capacity Development and Hygiene Measures in Yemen" and jointly implemented by Institute for Research in International Assistance (IRIA), and The Yemeni Association for Quality of Health Services and Development (YAQHSD)

AUTHOR

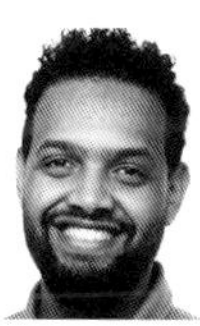

Alaaddin Alqadsi
Research Associate, Institute for Research in International Assistance (IRIA),
Akkon Hochschule für Humanwissenschaften, Berlin, Germany
E-mail: Alaaddin.Alqadsi@iria.akkon-hochschule.de

#12.1 *Conference Report*
A conference report to the World Health Summit 2022
Jean-Philippe L.D.S. Stolte

KEYWORD. One Health Strategy, Global Health

INTRODUCTION. The World Health Summit (WHS) joins forces for the first time with the World Health Organization (WHO) to host the international conference in Berlin from the 16th to the 18th of October 2022. Where experts working in science, politics, non-Governmental Organisations, people from the public and private sectors and from around the world come together to learn from the Covid 19 Pandemic and prepare for future crises. Maintaining a close eye on Global Health and Health Systems, the WHS promotes open discussions and critical debates of the highest level.
Concentrating on the program of the 16th of October. The Workshop "One Voice for a European Global Health and One Health Strategy" which aims to adapt and strengthen the European global health policy strategy, to better align with One Health priorities and the Sustainable Development Goals (SDGs) while also rethinking international cooperation.

INTRODUCTION STATEMENT. The Moderator Benoît Miribel Secretary-General of the One sustainable Health for all Foundation in France, reflects in his introduction speech on the crucial needs of a unified health policy.
He refers to the updated European Global Health Strategy which should enable an integrated and complementary decision process by European member states and multilateral organizations. It should also outline how to establish equal partnerships, especially with an eye on the global south.
Furthermore, the mission of One Europe for Global Health (OEGH) follows the Lyon Declaration which was signed on February 8th, 2022. With the intention of improving and integrating Global Health and One Health priorities into European policies, strategies, and actions. This will be done through the engagement of European civil society and actors from every sector.
He then finishes his introduction with the statement that we all share a common responsibility for the future generation. That the OEGH stands for the future generation and that we must act locally while thinking globally. To achieve an effective governance, we must work together in equity.

1. Speaker. As the first speaker Rhoda Wanyenz, who is the Dean of the Makerere University School of Public Health in Uganda, takes on the podium to give perspectives on health issues in the global south. She mentions the past experiences of the Covid-19 Pandemic and other crises like climate change and antimicrobial resistance that have taken place during that time. Have shown that it is not just about health. We need to look beyond the Health sector and include the Ecosystem, the Animals, the environment and everything that is in it in the concept of One Health. She stressed the importance of collaboration for a One European Health, which can only be reached through a Global Health, and vice versa. She then carries on and empathises on 4 Key issues that must be acknowledged for it to work:

(1) To adapt Global Health to the needs of each country because not every key fits into every lock. Due to a lack of devotion over the past 2 years, many Women and Children have died due to other causes than the Covid-Pandemic in Africa. The One Health Strategy must therefore be more relevant to each health system, to for example be able to withstand the simultaneous outbreak of multiple diseases in Africa.

(2) Investing in Data and Research to drive action: Without data, there can be no action. Therefore an investment in data and the means to analyse it must be made on a local and global scale to then be used as guidance.

(3) Equalities: In order to fully participate in the ecosystem for research and innovation, a special focus should be placed on SDG 10: reducing inequality. This is relevant to health determinants and intersects with sectors such as health access, education, technologies and skills. It also plays a major role in partnerships, where a mechanism should be established to deal with inequality so that it does not hinder solutions and innovation.

(4) Education systems: In order to create future changemakers and leaders for Sustainable One Health, education systems need to be adapted to focus on education, research, and innovation and seen as long term investments.

2. Speaker. Ole Petter Ottersen, who is the president of the Karolinska Institute in Sweeden, states during his presentation that the Lyon declaration puts Health in the centre stage in Europe and worldwide and is encompassed through 4 C's:

(1) Cooperation: that Cooperation isn't limited to Europe, but also extends beyond, and we need a global perspective. He also makes it clear that we do not need self-reliance and self-sufficiency since we are all connected.

(2) Convergence: Priorities must be linked and connected to major health problems.

(3) Context: Future policies must take the health of animals and the planet into account.

(4) Cross-sectorial interdisciplinary approach to health: Government that is for health and takes into account that health is impacted and generated throughout all sectors of society.

He adds a final C for Consistency: the continued work in this field.

3. Speaker. As the next speaker Karin R. Spido, who is a professor of medicine

#12.1 Conference Report
A conference report to the World Health Summit 2022

and head of Experimental Cardiology at the Catholic University in Leuven takes the podium. She presents concepts devolved in the scientific Panel for health with a focus on the Question: Is health research in the European Union fit for purpose? In the first slide of her PowerPoint presentation, she compares Health and Health research in EU treaties. She explains that Health is not one of the main competences of the European treaty, but it does engage itself in a high-level protection of Human Health. Member states oversee their own National Health services and medical support while the EU supports those activities. Furthermore, while engagement in setting up agencies has been evident, the financial support behind it has not. Whereas the investment in research as a main competence has been vigorously supported. Examining the content of the health research programmes in the EU multi-annual framework, where every 7-year priorities are set and instruments are developed to implement these. Many instruments can be identified. Despite this, she empathizes on the keyword: fragmentation. Fragmentation that spreads into funding, because EU-level funding for health research in 2020 is 1.3 billion, but in the member states, it was 19 billion and although the member states have greater funding, they lack the power of collaborative research, which the EU is known for. In her next slide, the EU health research spending of the year 2019 is displayed in comparison to the rest of the world. While the DFG from Germany and INERM from France support research in the EU, other countries like Japan and Canada are comparable to them, despite being a single funding agency. Moreover, they represent only a fraction of what the NIH ifrom the US spends. In her last slide, she stresses that a lot of European countries do not have a dedicated Health Program. Thus a strong guidance for a health research strategy is needed in the European Health Union. Yet in order for the EU to speak on a global scale, it requires a well-functioning government within the EU, that combines all of the available components under a strong leadership. Strong cooperation between stakeholders and a similar leadership style to that of the US is essential for an acknowledgable European Health Union.

4. Speaker. As the next speaker Michael Kazatchkine, who is an advisor of the Joint United Nations Programme on HIV/AIDS (UNAIDS) and speaks on behalf of Santé Mondiale 2030 makes 3 Points in his speech.

(1) Maintaining political momentum for global health through the lessons learned from the Covid Pandemic and the recurring EU Global halth Strategy. Because on a global level, health has shifted from a simple agenda to a critical economic and security issue. Which has been the main topic at the G7, G20 and WTO ministerial meetings. Additionally, there will be three high-level meetings at the UN General Assembly about global health in 2023.

(2) An external European agenda for health is just as necessary as an internal European agenda for health. For the one health approach to work, one voice in global health must exist and The One Voice must be based on the values of solidarity, support for resilient health systems, commitment to equity, inclusivity, multilateralism, and commitment to sustainable development.

(3) There must be clear guidance regarding the appliance of one health and a structure of priorities that must be agreed on together to achieve the greatest impact.

Kazatchkine mentions 4 areas to invest in One Health. **(1)** Anti-microbial resistance.
(2) Enhancing health surveillance systems.
(3) refocus Europe's cooperation investment in research, capacity building and emerging infectious disease hotspot countries like Africa.
(4) A joint European action and a greater degree of coordination.

5. Speaker. On the podium, Clément Martin Auer, who is the President of the European Health Forum Gastein in Austria, makes 3 points, as well.

In his **(1)** key point he mentions that he feels as if he would be in a déjà vu because 20 years ago there was already the idea of a Global Health Strategy, that faded into existence and has now resurfaced.

In his **(2)** key point, he explains that the EU, in particular, the European Commission with its 27 member states, is a global player whose members want to strengthen multilateralism.

He expressed that it was the EU who pushed through to create an intergovernmental negotiation Process, that would produce new legally binding instruments for better prevention and preparedness of public health catastrophes.

He then moves on to his final keypoint. It focuses on the delighted events that led to a convergence between global strategy thinking and global health thinking, in which he argues that every nation should participate more actively in political discussions. Moreover, the image of charity needs to change to one of cooperative empowerment protected by investments.

6. Speaker. Heilia Agueda Molina Milman, who is a member of the Chilian Parlament, discusses in her speach how to better align the European and Global health strategy with the One Health priorities and Sustainable Development Goals in Latin American and Caribbean countries.

She suggests 5 priorities to collaboratively and integratively work together with the EU.

#12.1 Conference Report
A conference report to the World Health Summit 2022

(1) In order to achieve universal health coverage and to ensure no one is left behind, she emphasized the need for improving health systems. To address health and equality and ensure social protection in health. She continius with the fact that Europe has already achieved this and that they should share their lessons learned and good practices.
(2) A more effective and flexible way is needed to trade related aspects of intellectual property rights, to close the gap in research and innovation.
(3) Addressing health inequalities and the social determinants of health. Where gaps in terms of income capacity, productivity and access to public goods must be closed.
(4) Environmental factors and climate change. We must create new mechanisms to finance sustainable investments that address both global health and climate change.
(5) Strong leadership in Global Health diplomacy and a better global government is needed, to strengthen multilateralism beyond the European borders.
(6) The European Union and Latin American Caribbean must strengthen their strategic partnership because no one can face the aftermath of the Covid Pandemic alone.

7. Speaker. Alena Šteflová, who will speak on behalf of the Czech medical association and the Czech Presidency at the EU to outline the contribution of the Czech presidency.
She clarifies that it is in the interest of the Czech presidency to commit to communication and cooperation with the European Commission and the member states. To be able to implement unified European strategies, negotiations and voices must also exist. Where she refers to the WHS as the suitable place for it. In addition, meetings can be set up by the Czech presidency to discuss these topics. She empathizes that the Czech Presidency has very clear goals regarding European health issues and that the gatherings could still be access points for discussions. She remarks that under the Czech presidency, the Prague declaration on synergies in the research and innovation funding in Europe has already been adopted. According to her, these points could be relevant for the Lyon declaration and could resolve fragmentation issues. Furthermore, she emphasizes the importance of the concept of diversity and that bridges should be built instead of trenches between states.
She goes on to say that although there is a history between the states and that they are diverse, that influences healthcare delivery systems, economic development, and political positions. The recent historical situation is more critical than ever and a change in attitudes and opinions is needed between countries for a better future.

8. Speaker. John F. Ryan, who is the deputy director general of health and food

safety at the EU commission, expresses his viewpoints to the Panel.
He begins with a standpoint of the EU internal policies from the EU perspective. He outlines that One Health is not a new concept, it has just been rising up again due to the Covid pandemic. Besides the Covid pandemic, there are silent pandemics such as Zika in Africa, but the link between human health, animal health, and plant health is the key.
Therefore, the Commission fully supports the 2021 definition of One Health: an integrated unifying approach that aims to sustainable balance and optimize the health of people, animals and ecosystems.
From the perspective of antimicrobial resistance which affects animal health, the use of pharmaceuticals and human health. where as Human health lies in the responsibilities of the member state, whereas the responsibilities for animal health and the use of pharmaceuticals lie at a European level. The legal situation therefore is complex and is currently being simplified through a more balanced and rational approach, considering the antimicrobial resistance concept in a more integrated way. Which can only be achieved through integrated surveillance and surveillance systems, which depend on a digital Europe and digital health.
The second approach that is to be adopted is strengthening the agencies and the strengthening of legislations on cross-border threats. Which should lead to a better detection and response system for issues like antimicrobial resistance. He continues that through an integrated response, the committees of member states could come together and involve all the different sectors or areas. The difficulty lies in the implementation of this multisectoral approach because legislations are often outdated and have to be adapted to current knowledge.
This is similar to research, which should have a forward-looking agenda to identify future problems. In his final point, he describes the EU's approach to health-related policies. Which involves the reform of the common agricultural policy, which links agricultural production to the health agenda. Like for example the issue of red meat and the use of dairy products and their health benefits.
During his last remarks, he referred to the Global health strategy, which he stated would bridge the gap between the SDGs, global health needs, and our domestic policies to promote a multinational approach to global health.

9. Speaker. Ffion Storer Jones, who is an advocate officer at the German Foundation for World Population (DSW) and represents an NGO that is part of the coalition and will focus on human health and human rights.
She proceeded to give an overview of the need to connect advocacy efforts to policy and will focus on the new EU's global health strategy and its im-

plementation. She explained that the EU's framework is outdated in crucial areas like antimicrobial resistance, sexual reproductive health and rights and pandemic preparedness. Afterwards, she criticized the Framework for lacking any monitoring structure or dedicated budget, which made it impossible to evaluate its impact. She then changes her position and explains, that despite those arguments, the DWS is delighted to see that the EU strategy is in consultation and incorporates low- and middle-income countries in the new strategy. After that, she outlines 3 points that the DWS proposes to make this Strategy successful.

(1) Research and development for updated and improved tools, to decrease the impact of the climate crisis on people's health. This includes sexual and reproductive health, rising threats of epidemics and infectious diseases and similar AMR.

(2) Policies are not enough and they need to be backed up by a robust funding framework. She explains that while the UK and the US dedicate 15%-30% of their official budgets to health, the EU only dedicated 5%. Therefore, an increase in global health funding is necessary.

(3) Commitments and principles must be followed by actions, to be impactful. A strategic framework with a detailed implementation plan and a robust monitoring and evaluation framework, which includes measurable, relevant indicators for reporting progress, is imperative. She concludes her speech with the mark that through the involvement of local CSOs, communities, citizens, people in parliament and other stakeholders, a successful design of health programs can be created, and through further involvement of civil society and other stakeholders, advocacy can become policy, and policy becomes impact.

QUESTIONS AND ANSWERS. As a first reaction to the discussion the Moderator askes Stéphanie Seydoux, the French ambassador for Global Health, for a reaction. In her reaction she states that a few key points have been made clear. All the voices from the different fields, representing different regions of the world, are in sync and have a shared vision of a One Global Health.

She also mentions that Europe has a great opportunity to play this role. This is as long as it manages to seize the moment and overcome the complex challenges that have been mentioned. Furthermore, Europe has a chance because its vision of health is imbedded into its values.

As second reactor to the discussion, the Moderator invites Dr. Anders Nordström, the Swedish ambassador for global health, to the podium.in his speech he outlines that the current EU strategies are based on the Millennium Development Goals and that despite its positive impact on the world, times have changed, especially since the Covid pandemic. The new strategy therefore needs to address 3 components.

(1) how we will be able to have a safer world and better prepare and respond

(2) continue the work of enabling access to basic health service for everybody regardless of ability to pay universal health coverage

(3) Need to invest in preventive measures, such as what we eat.

The second change that needs to be made is the implementation of the strategy. While the old strategy was based on AId paradigm, the new strategy should be based on equal partnerships on equal terms.

THANK YOU SPEECH. The Moderator thanks all the speakers and all the participants and invites Detlev Ganten, The president of the World health Summit to the podium to hold a closing Speech. In his Statement he wants to highlight that the real challenge lies in overcoming complexity in the Global world.

Additionally, these events should aim to find a person with a specific amount of charisma for a topic in order to create an impact and then be supported through everybody else. He finishes his speech with the key words: Overcome Complexity through Simplicity.—

AUTHOR

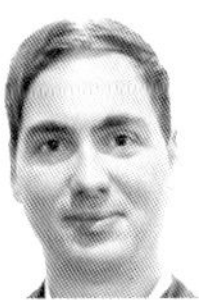

Jean-Philippe L.D.S. Stolte
Student International Emergency and Disaster Relief
Akkon Hochschule für Humanwissenschaften, Berlin, Germany
E-mail: j.philippe.stolte@gmail.com

#12.2 Conference Report Report from World Health Summit, Berlin, Germany – sexual and reproductive health and rights for all

Laura Schlucke

In this workshop, the main topic of the very interesting participants was "Ensuring Access to Services as Part of UHC [universal health coverage] and Resilient Health Systems". Many interesting participants added their expertise to this topic, with much discussion about the impact of Covid-s 19 pandemic. Unfortunately, the pandemic had set back many promising projects and pushed many health systems to the limits of their capacity. It also set back progress in the Sexual Reproductive health and Rights (SRHR) sector, including Maternal, Newborn and Child Heath (MNCH). An equally important point is "Health for all", which stands as a guiding principle of UHC and could only be implemented if a human rights-based approach is realized that includes all people, marginalized as well as furthest left behind.

In order to give an insight into the different topics discussed, a brief summary of several important interventions follows.

First and foremost, Natalia Kanem, Director of the UNFPA, emphasized right at the beginning that health and access to health systems should not be a luxury, but a human right. This access must also be accompanied by a certain quality of care, because the extent to which women cannot give birth safely or do not have access to trained midwives is very serious. Usually, the people who already have the least suffer the most from a poor health care system. In addition, he said, the empowerment of women cannot be divorced from this discussion – they must be included in decision-making processes and also seen as an integral part of family planning.

Awa Marie Coll Seck, Minister of State of the Presidency of Senegal, also stressed that, especially in international programs, countries must be in the drivers seat to ensure success. In Senegal, the Covid-19 pandemic has been particularly hard on people working in the front line and has destabilized the health system for the long term. This also led to the halting of some international programs, such as the HPV vaccination programs, to the detriment of many women. These would only now have to be restarted, costing a lot of precious time.

Bärbel Kofler, Parliamentary State Secretary to the Federal Minister for Economic Cooperation and Development (BMZ), stressed the importance of access to a health system that covers basic needs, even in the most remote areas of the world. Therefore, the BMZ puts at the center of their work to support projects and organizations, also with large financial resources, that address this major issue.

Sahar Al Qawasmi, member of Palestinian Legislative Council, added that this issue can not go without the point genderequality, because access must be equal and characterized by free choices. In summary, participants from Zambia, presented as "young voices", who were connected online, summed it up: decisions must be made freely and self-determined, must be affordable and, in the best case, freely available, must be part of education in schools, and the infrastructure must be in place. It is equally important to pay attention to the mental health of young people and to make no distinction between "normal" health and reproductive health.—

AUTHOR

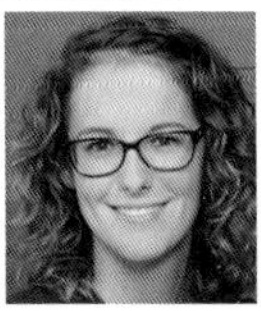

Laura Schlucke
Student International Emergency and Disaster Relief
Akkon Hochschule für Humanwissenschaften, Berlin, Germany
laura.schlucke@t-online.de

Koch Metschnikow Forum

Koch-Mechnikov Forum (KMF) is a German-Eastern European scientific non-governmental non-commercial organisation active in healthcare realm. It was established in 2006 with the purpose of contributing to aligning the Eastern European healthcare systems with the German healthcare. The legal framework along with the guiding priorities for its activities are enshrined in the Eastern Partnership Initiative of the German government.

For over ten years, KMF has been implementing a wide range of projects and activities such as organization of conferences, seminars, research stays, and other forms of medical and scientific exchange. Hitherto, it has successfully carried out over 150 projects on different medical topics together with its partner organisations from Russia (until Feb. 2022!), Georgia, Belarus and Moldova. Health ministries, research institutes, medical universities, health service providers, professional associations, diverse representatives of civil society, and pharmaceutical companies with *social responsibility* form a broad network of KMF. The work is carried out in different sections, whose heads are reknown experts in their specific medicine-related fields. The main office located in the old historical building *LangenbeckVirchow House* in the Berlin downtown is responsible for general coordination of projects and cross-sectional activities.

You can send requests to:

Prof. Dr. med. Helmut Hahn
President of Koch-Metschnikow-Forum e.V.,
Langenbeck-Virchow-Haus
Luisenstraße 59
10117 Berlin, Germany

E-Mail: hahn@kmforum.de